MW00714865

fit for life

FITNESS
FOR WOMEN

Credits:

Art Director: Peter Bridgewater
Editorial Consultants: Maria Pal/Clark Robinson Ltd
Photography: Paul Forrester, assisted by John Alflatt
Model: Catherine Mackwood

Picture credits:

key: r = right

The author and publishers have made every effort to identify the
copyright owners of the photographs; they apologize for any
omissions and wish to thank the following:

David Burch, 7, 70, 72r, 77; Richard and Sally Greenhill, 71;
TWA Getaway Club, 81; The Wool Bureau, 83.

fit for life

FITNESS
FOR WOMEN

K A R E N   L I P T A K

Gallery Books
an imprint of W.H. Smith Publishers, Inc.
112 Madison Avenue, New York
New York 10016

A QUARTO BOOK

This edition published in 1990 by Gallery Books,
an imprint of W.H. Smith Publishers, Inc.,
112, Madison Avenue, New York, New York 10016

Gallery Books are available for bulk purchase for
sales promotions and premium use. For details write or
telephone the Manager of Special Sales, W.H. Smith
Publishers Inc., 112 Madison Avenue, New York, New
York 10016. (212) 532-6600.

ISBN 0-8317-3892-8

The information and recommendations contained in this book
are intended to complement, not substitute for, the advice of
your own physician. Before starting any medical treatment,
exercise program or diet, consult your physician. Information is
given without any guarantees on the part of the author and
publisher, and they cannot be held responsible for the contents
of this book.

► CONTENTS

EXERCISE . . . AND ENJOY LIFE MORE   6

WORKING UP TO WORKING OUT   8

WARM-UPS   10

HIP EXERCISES   16

THIGH EXERCISES   21

BUST EXERCISES   26

UPPER ARM EXERCISES   31

BUTTOCK EXERCISES   36

WAIST EXERCISES   41

STOMACH EXERCISES   45

COOL-DOWN EXERCISES   50

PRENATAL SHAPE-UP   55

PRENATAL EXERCISES   56

BAD BACK REPORT   60

BACK EXERCISES   62

SLIMMING ON THE SLY   64

WEIGHT TRAINING   66

AEROBICS . . . A HEALTH PHENOMENON   70

MONITOR YOUR PROGRESS   71

THREE AEROBIC FAVORITES: 72
    JOGGING, WALKING, DANCING

NUTRIENTS, THE BASIC   74
    FOUR + ONE, AND YOU

HEALTHY FOOD HABITS   76

THE DANGER OF DIETS   77

THE WORST DIETARY OFFENDERS   78

EATING OUT WITHOUT GUILT   80

POSTURE POINTERS   82

BREATHING FOR FITNESS   84

QUESTIONS ABOUT EXERCISE AND DIET   85

PROGRESS REPORT   90

INDEX   94

▶ EXERCISE... AND ENJOY LIFE MORE

Every woman wants to look her best, and it's no secret that exercise, when combined with a healthy diet, helps you do just that. Those pounds we put on from overindulging ourselves in life's technological labor-saving devices and culinary goodies have a way of not only making us look less fit, but also of leaving us feeling less up to par.

A planned combination of exercise and sensible eating can do wonders for your physical well-being, and your psyche as well. Even if you weigh your optimum weight, you still need a regular routine of workouts to keep your body firm and strong, rather than weak and flabby.

A steady exercise program gets you in condition to deal with the trials and tribulations, the ups and downs, the inevitable stresses, as well as the joys, of daily life. Whether your work is at home, at an office, or on the road, exercise done regularly gives you the energy you need to get your tasks done efficiently, and still have plenty of charge left in your battery to enjoy everything else life has to offer.

If you've put off regular exercising and weight watching, you're not alone. Millions of excuses exist for people looking for reasons to procrastinate starting what is paramount to a new lifestyle. But once you get into the "slim of things", you'll wonder why you put it off for so long. With perseverance to get through your first few days, the results you'll soon see and feel will fortify your determination to make this your new way of life.

Exercise has many benefits going for it!

You'll keep your weight in check, reduce your risk of diabetes, gallstones, osteoarthritis and circulatory diseases. You'll help prevent arthritis and osteoporosis (thinning of the bones). You gain all this, besides looking healthier, sleeping sounder, feeling calmer, having clearer skin, more lustrous hair, and an improved outlook on life. So, let your desire to live the best life you can be the chief motivator to improve . . . by starting to move. And join the millions who have crossed over the line from inactivity to activity.

This valuable guide can help you get started. Its handy size means you can easily carry it with you wherever you go. Turn to its exercises often. They're designed to tone and condition the parts of a woman's body that most need firming. While different exercises emphasize different trouble spots, each exercise generally works on a whole area of your body, so that you achieve overall shape-up results.

Of course, exercise isn't the only factor affecting your positive enjoyment of life. But it is undeniably a major one. So, get into your exercise mode, put your body in gear, and make this your fitness year.

To begin, look in the mirror. Decide how you want to look three months from now, six months, a year. Don't expect miracles overnight. That only leads to disappointments. A steady, consistent shaping-up and conditioning is your most realistic goal.

Then, go at it! Work alone, or round up your friends for an exercise and diet support group. But, by all means, whether you have your friends' comraderie or not, start enhancing your life with exercise today!

Make a commitment to exercise and stick with it. Remember, nobody will take you by the hand and lead you to exercise and to devise a diet plan right for you. *You've* got to take that first step. Once you do, the rest follows. Rather than look at what exercise might take away from you (an extra half hour of sleep in the morning, or rest before dinner), concentrate instead on how much a good exercise program will bring into your life.

The odds are definitely in favor of exercising. They tip the good-living scale in your favor. C'mon! Join the millions of women who've found that a commitment to fitness pays off. Get into the swing, the sway, the twist, and the lunge of things.

Exercise . . . and get into shape for the rest of a wonderful life.

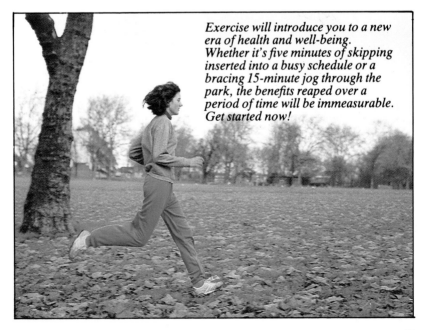

Exercise will introduce you to a new era of health and well-being. Whether it's five minutes of skipping inserted into a busy schedule or a bracing 15-minute jog through the park, the benefits reaped over a period of time will be immeasurable. Get started now!

▶ WORKING UP TO WORKING OUT

You may want to compensate for a long stretch of inactivity by plunging into a full-scale exercise program. Please don't. The best way to start your muscles working again after long periods of underutilization is *gradually*. Start with as little as five minutes a day of exercise. Work up to 10 minutes, then 15-, 20-, and 30-minute sessions. Be sure to include warm-ups and cool-downs in your exercise schedule. They are for your protection, as well as fitness.

WARM-UPS

When you warm up, you increase your body temperature and heart beat, opening up your blood vessels in preparation for the extra pumping of blood you'll soon require. Warm-ups also help you maintain flexibility, which becomes even more important as you get older, and your tissues lose their youthful elasticity, and exhibit a greater tendency to strain. Injuries are often caused by neglecting this initial stage of your exercise routine.

MAIN EXERCISES

A variety of exercises to tighten up your muscles all over your body are given in the main section of this guide. Choose an assortment from each section so you don't overindulge one area of your body and wind up with new bulges, rather than the sleek all-over figure you're seeking.

COOL-DOWNS

After your main exercises, blood may collect in areas of your body you've worked on, especially in your legs. By doing cool-down exercises, you taper off gradually, and give your blood the time it needs to return to your overall circulation.

We suggest three exercise periods a week for beginners. On alternate days your body has a chance to rest and recuperate from the new activity you've awakened it to.

Eventually, exercise will become a way of life with you, and you'll want to alternate toning exercises with aerobic exercises. The back of this book provides you with the aerobic lowdown and helps you work out a routine that is both enjoyable, effective and beneficial for you.

WORKING UP TO WORKING OUT

EXERCISE TIPS

Here are some tips to help you shape up smartly from the start.

- **Music to exercise by.** No need for exercise to be a dreary time of day. Keep your exercise periods something to anticipate with pleasure. Turning on the music is one way to get your body moving. Or you might try exercising to your favorite TV shows.
- **When to exercise.** Choose a special time, and try sticking to it each day. That way you'll create an exercise habit your body will get used to. When you miss your allotted time, you'll consciously know something's not right. Experts agree that almost any time is good, except you are cautioned not to exercise right before going to sleep, and not within an hour after eating a meal.
- **What to wear.** Dress comfortably. Lucky you. Times have changed from the days of the traditional black leotard. Now you're free to exercise in a variety of pretty clothes that allow you to move around without restriction. Just remember to keep whatever you're wearing loose.
- **Ventilate the area.** When it's not too cold out, keep a window open, so you get plenty of air. The more oxygen in the room, the more energy you'll have. If the air's brisk outside, but feels refreshing you may want to compensate by dressing with added layers of loose clothing that you can remove as necessary.
- **Where to exercise.** Make sure you've got plenty of room, so your leg kicks and arm stretches don't destroy the furniture or you. For floor exercises, choose an area that's got soft carpeting, or else pull a scatter rug, mat, or blanket over a hard floor.
- **Breathe!** Sounds simple enough, but sometimes it isn't. Many people make the mistake of thinking that they shouldn't breathe while exercising. *Always breathe when you exercise.* The preferred breathing pattern is to breath in on each effort you make, and breathe out on each relaxation. See the back of this book for more information on proper breathing and its benefits.
- **Expect slight soreness.** If you haven't exercised regularly for a while, don't be surprised to feel slightly sore when you first get started. This is your muscles' way of protesting a change. However, beware if you suffer from any real physical pain or excessive fatigue. In either case, stop your routine immediately.
- **Drink when thirsty.** Dehydration can lead to problems. If you're thirsty before, during, or after exercising, don't hesitate to drink cool or lukewarm water. (Iced water can cause cramps.)
- **Hot showers.** Never take a hot shower or bath right after exercising. Always wait until you've cooled down sufficiently.
- *Always consult with your doctor before beginning this or any exercise program. Then proceed with your physician's approval or with medical restrictions in mind.*

▶ *WARM-UPS*

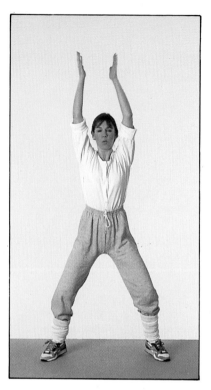

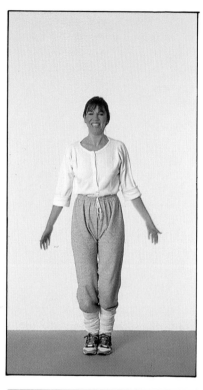

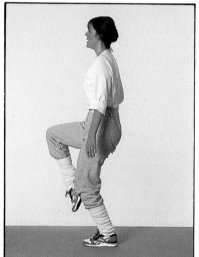

WARM-UP #1

Jump out while clapping
your hands above your head.

Then jump back in, slapping
hands at thighs. Start with 10
repetitions (10X). Gradually
increase to 25 repetitions (25X).

WARM-UP #2

LEFT: Run in place at an easy
pace with your elbows bent and
freely swinging at your waist
level. Count to 10. Gradually
increase to 50.

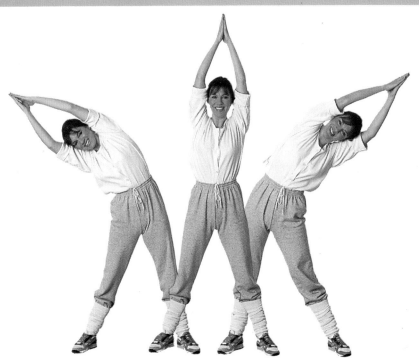

Stand straight, feet slightly apart, palms touching above head.

With elbows straight, palms pressed together, bend from waist to one side.

Return and bend to other side. Do 10X.

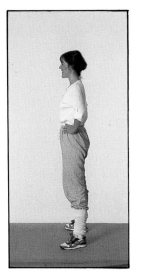

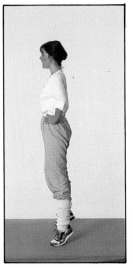

Stand straight, feet slightly apart, hands on hips.

Raise heels off floor, then lower. Do 25X. Gradually increase to 50X.

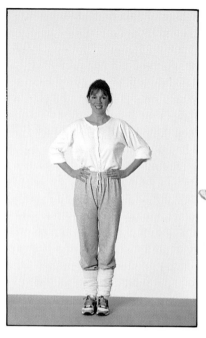

WARM-UP #5

Stand straight, elbows flexed, weight on toes.

Kick out one foot to side and back. Do same with other foot. Do 10X each side.

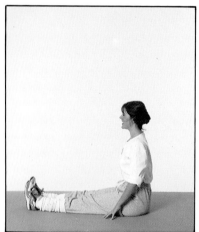

WARM-UP #6

Sit on floor with both legs straight in front, arms at side.

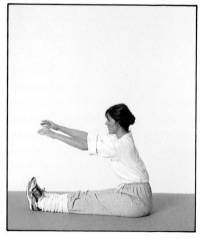

Lift arms overhead and reach down to toes. Hold for count of 5, return to start and do 10X.

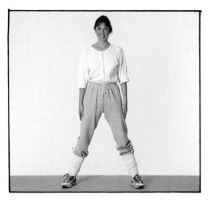

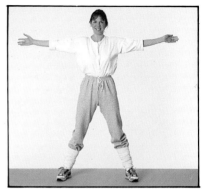

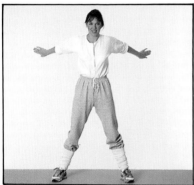

WARM-UP #7

Stand straight with feet wide apart.

Lift arms up, palms forward, then to side.

Swing arms back, with palms back. Hold for count of 5 in each position. Do 10X.

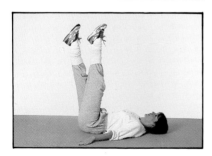

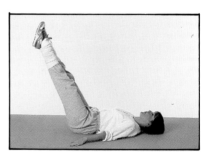

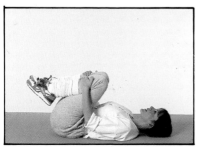

WARM-UP #8

Lie flat on floor with hands at sides, palms down and lift feet straight up.
Slowly lower them while criss-crossing in scissors movement. Bring knees into chest with hands. Then start again. Do 6X to begin. Work up to 10X.

Lie on your right side, with your right hand supporting your head, and your left hand in front of you on the floor.

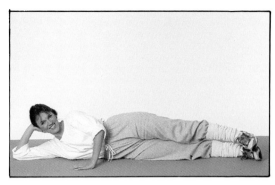

With legs straight and together, raise your left leg straight up as far as possible. Lower. Do 10X each side.

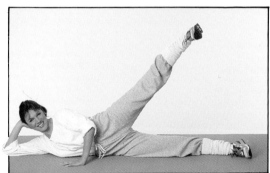

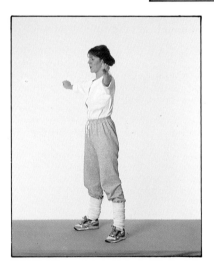

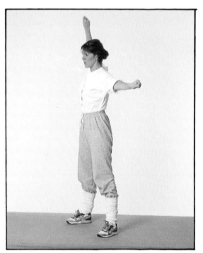

Stand straight with feet moderately separated and arms stretched out.

Make large backward circles with them, moving one at a time. Do 10X each arm.

14

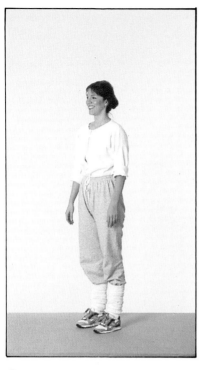

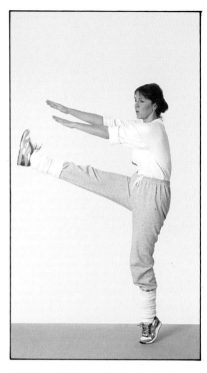

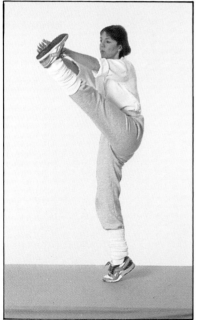

WARM-UP #11

Stand straight, hands loose at sides.

While hopping on one leg, kick other up and out and try to touch its toes with both hands.

Do 10X each leg.

▶ *HIP EXERCISES*

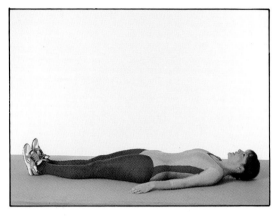

Lie on floor, legs together, arms flat at sides.

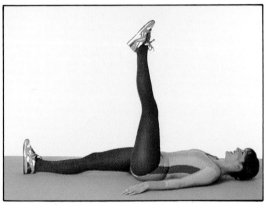

Lift one leg straight up as high as possible and make 10 wide circles clockwise, then 10 counterclockwise. Keep toes pointed.

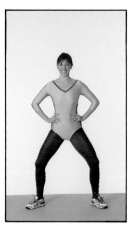 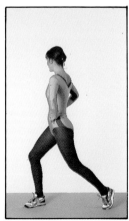

Stand, elbows bent, knees slightly flexed, heels raised.

Twist hips, arms, heels in same direction. Then opposite direction. Do 20 repetitions (20X).

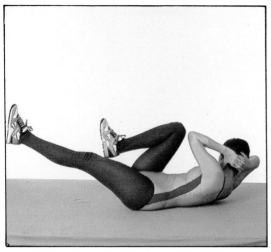

Lie on floor, legs straight ahead, toes pointed and hands behind head. Twist upper body to bring right knee up to touch left elbow.

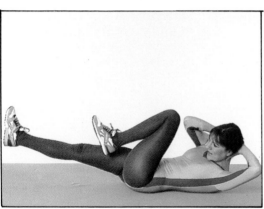

Return to start and alternate breathing out as you do exercise and pull stomach muscles in.

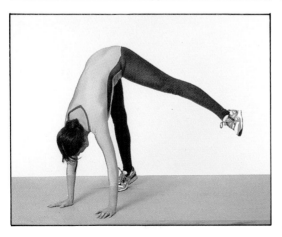

Bend over, palms flat on floor, right leg straight, and left leg extended out to left side. Raise up right heel and left leg at same time. Return to start. Alternate sides. Do 10X each side.

17

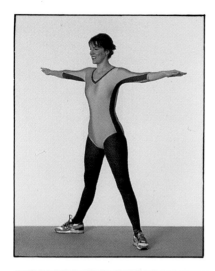

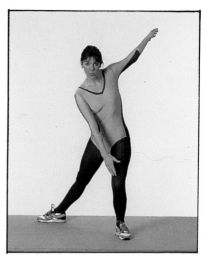

HIPS #5

Legs a giant step apart, toes out to sides, as are arms, and leaning slightly forward with knees flexed.

Straighten right knee as you rock body and right hand toward left. Alternate rock. Do 10X each side.

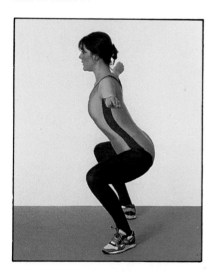

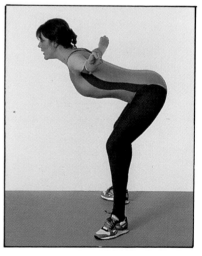

HIPS #6

Squat with toes out toward sides, and arms stretched straight out from shoulders.

With feet firm on floor, and knees bent, raise and lower hips. Do 20X.

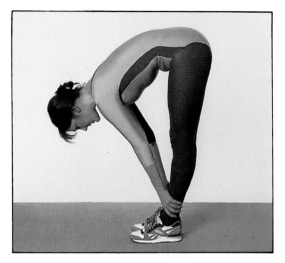

HIPS #7

Drop upper body forward and hold ankles with hands.

Straighten right leg as you bend left knee, turn left toes out, and sway to left. Alternate sides.

Do 10X each side.

HIPS #8

Rest on your elbows, with feet straight on floor. Bicycle legs straight up to count of 25. Gradually increase to count of 50.

19

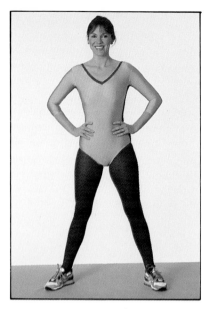 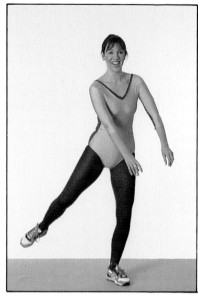

HIPS #9

Place hands on hips while standing with feet apart slightly.

Flex right knee, and hop on left foot while arms swing toward left. Do 10X. Then reverse action for 10X.

HIPS #10

Keep knees flexed as you lie on floor with arms near body, palms down.

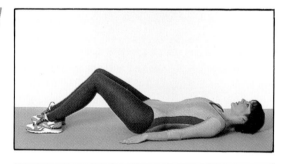

While keeping feet and shoulders on ground, lift hips from floor. Count to 5. Return to starting position. Do 10X.

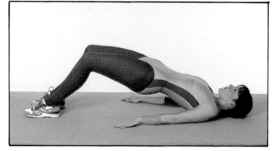

▶ THIGH EXERCISES

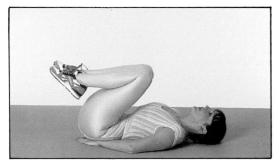

THIGHS #1

Lie on floor with hands under buttocks as support with knees bent into chest.

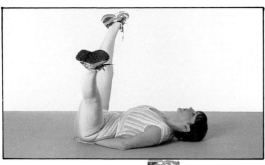

Lift legs straight up, open wide, and cross one over the other in a scissors movement to close them. Open and alternate. Do 10 repetitions (10X) open and close.

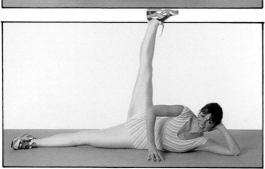

THIGHS #2

Lie on side, one hand supporting head, other supporting body in front.
Lift upper leg straight up in air.

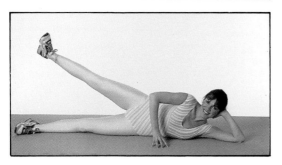

Then lower. Keep knee facing up. Do 10X each side.

THIGHS #3

Kneel on hands and knees with heels raised, and back flat.

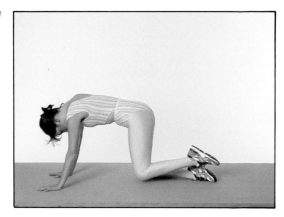

Thrust one leg straight out, forward and back. Keep knee straight. Do 10X. Switch sides. Do 10X more.

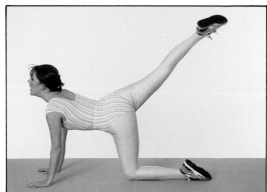

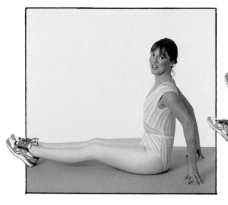

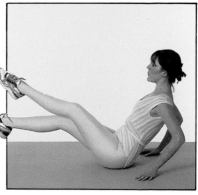

THIGHS #4

Sit with legs stretched ahead and place hands behind back for support.

Roll your pelvis back, raise both legs off the floor then cross one ankle in front of the other. Alternate. Do 10X.

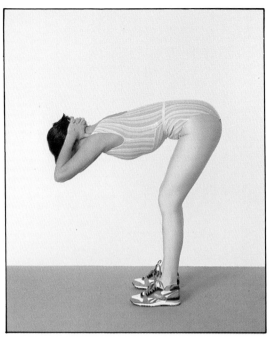

THIGHS #5.

Bend upper body toward floor, with hands clasped behind head, and elbows pointed down, knees slightly bent.

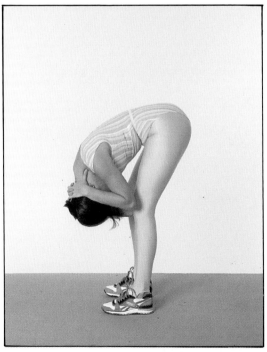

Twist upper body so both elbows reach left knee. (Bend of left leg will increase.) Do 15X each direction.

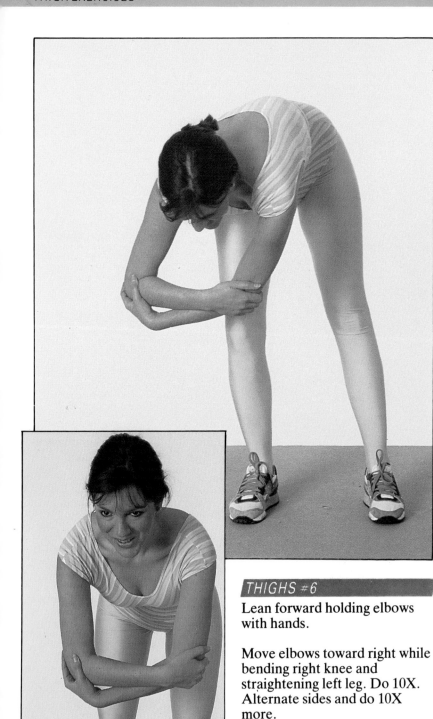

THIGHS #6

Lean forward holding elbows with hands.

Move elbows toward right while bending right knee and straightening left leg. Do 10X. Alternate sides and do 10X more.

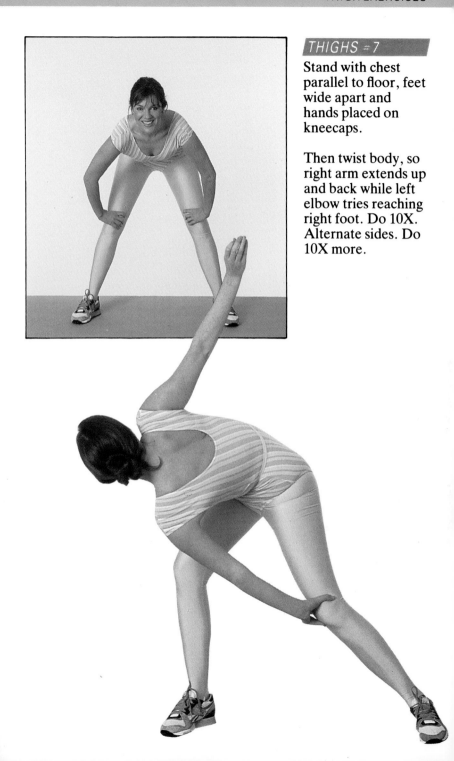

THIGHS ≠ 7

Stand with chest parallel to floor, feet wide apart and hands placed on kneecaps.

Then twist body, so right arm extends up and back while left elbow tries reaching right foot. Do 10X. Alternate sides. Do 10X more.

▶ *BUST EXERCISES*

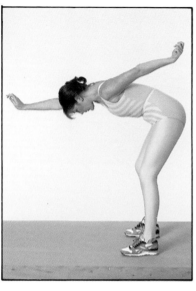

Bend forward and extend one arm straight back, the other straight ahead. Push back as hard as possible with arm in back. Reverse. Do 10 repetitions (10X) each arm.

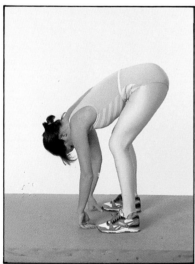

BUST #2

Drop upper body toward floor. Head down, arms loosely hanging.

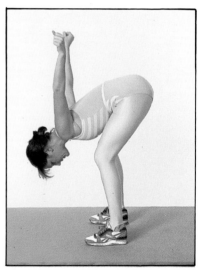

Bring arms up and back. Return to start position. Do 25X.

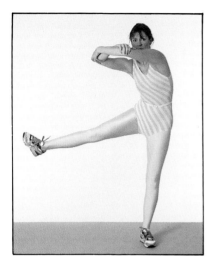

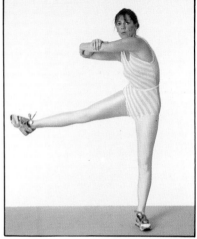

BUST #3

Stand with right leg stretched to side, and arms folded at eye level.

Raise right leg while moving elbows as far right as possible. Do 10X. Reverse. Do 10X more.

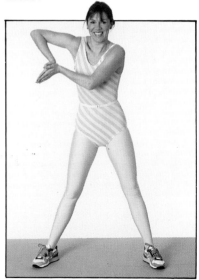

BUST #4

Stand with feet slightly apart, knees flexed, palms together, fingers down, elbows out at sides.

Swing elbows as far up as possible in swinging motion from one side to the other. Do 25X.

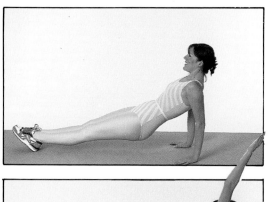

BUST #5

Sit on floor, and lean back with hands placed behind you. Then raise body slightly, with weight balanced on hands and heels.

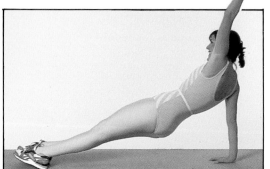

Lift up one arm as high as possible. Lower. Do 8X each side.

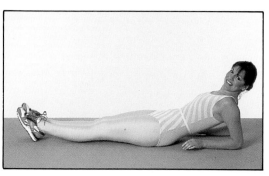

BUST #6

Sit on floor with legs straight ahead, and upper body raised. Rest on elbows.

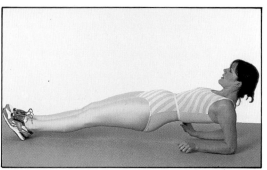

With elbows and heels remaining on ground, try raising body as high as possible. Lower. Do 20X.

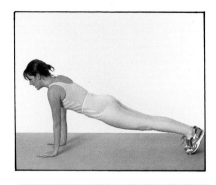

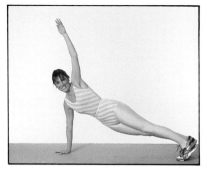

BUST #7

Put weight on hands and toes and keep arms and legs straight in push-up position.

Lift left arm and hips simultaneously. Lower. Alternate sides. Do 15X each side.

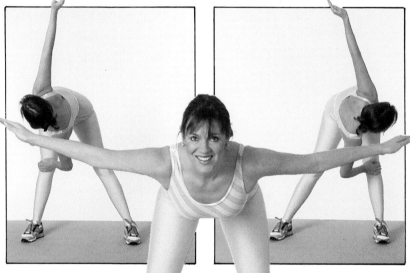

BUST #8

With arms stretched out at sides, lean forward from thighs.

Alternate sides. Do 20X each side.

Twist torso while bringing left arm down to right thigh, and lifting up right arm.

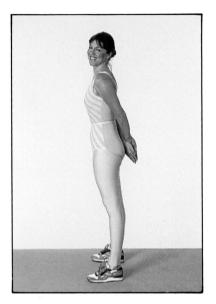

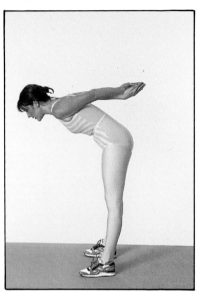

BUST #9

Place hands behind back at waist, left palm over right.

Bend forward. With palms still touching, bring hands up to shoulder-blade level, then lower to hips. Do 25X.

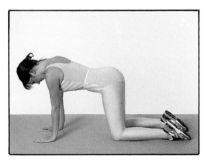

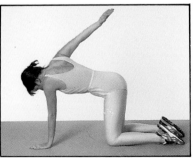

BUST #10

Kneel on hands and knees.

Lift one arm and bring across back, rotating it as you do so palm faces up.

Alternate sides. Do 10X each.

▶ *UPPER ARM EXERCISES*

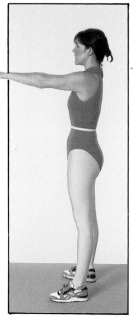 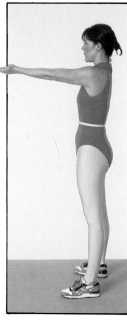

Stand straight, with arms stretched ahead at shoulder level, palms facing up.

Twist arms around so palms face down. Do 25 repetitions (25X).

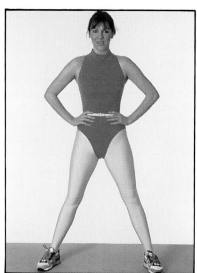 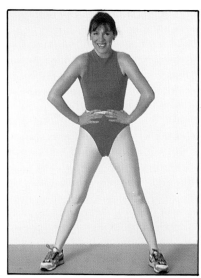

Feet wide apart, hands on waist.

Push elbows toward front, then back. Do 20X.

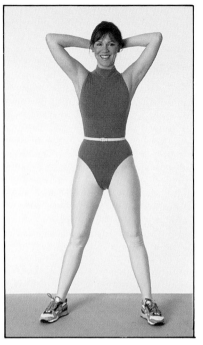

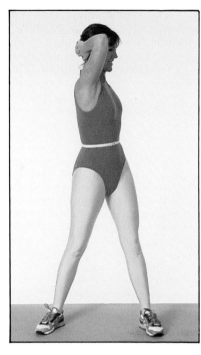

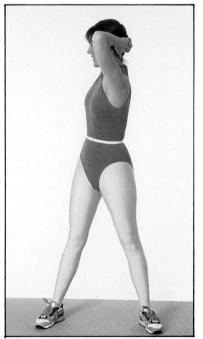

UPPER ARMS #3

Intertwine fingers behind head.

Twist elbows so one faces back, the other front.

Alternate sides. Do 20 twists.

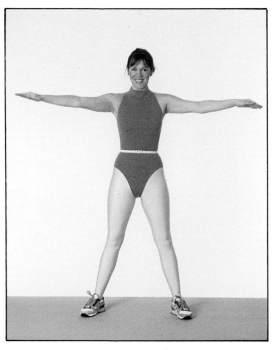

UPPER ARMS #4

Stand with feet slightly apart, arms straight out at sides.

Circle hands backward, then frontward. Do 5X each direction, 10 circles in all.

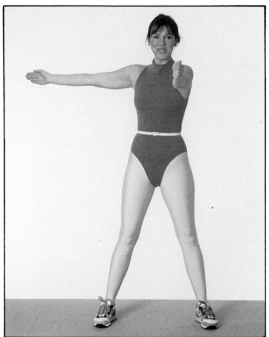

UPPER ARMS #5

Stand with feet apart, one arm stretched out straight ahead, the other out at side, both at shoulder level.

Cross body with arm stretched straight so it touches hand at side. Torso will twist with action. Alternate sides. Do 20X each side.

33

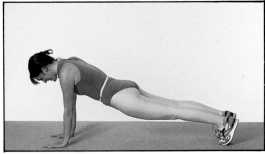

Balance on straight
arms and toes in
push-up position.

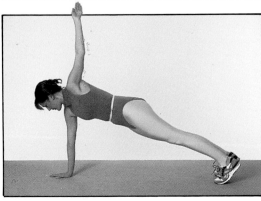

Raise one arm as far
up as possible.
Lower. Do 20X each
arm.

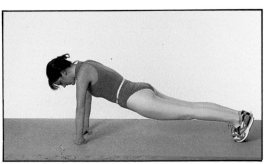

Balance on
straight arms and
toes in push-up
position once again.
This time, fingers
face each other.

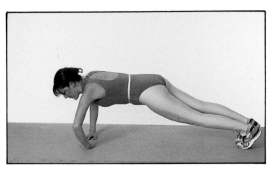

Flex one elbow until
it gets as close as
possible to floor. Do
5X each side.

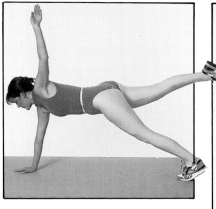

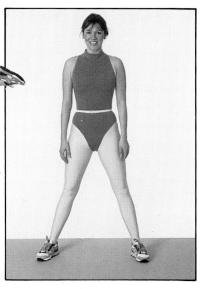

UPPER ARMS #8

Push-up position once again, arms and legs straight, hands and toes on floor. Raise opposite leg and arm as high as possible. Lower. Alternate sides. Do 20X.

UPPER ARMS #9

Stand with feet slightly apart, and hands hanging loosely down.

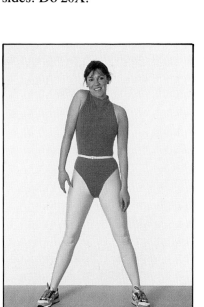

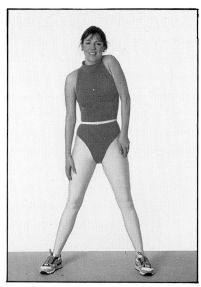

Raise one shoulder, then lower.

Repeat with other shoulder. Do 20X in all.

▶ *BUTTOCK EXERCISES*

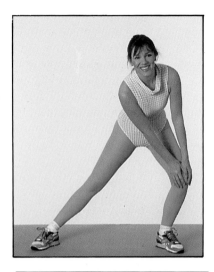 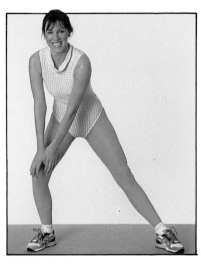

BUTTOCKS ≠1

Bend one knee while other leg is straight. Put both hands on bent knee. Hold for count of 10.

In a fluid movement, alternate sides. Hold for count of 10. Do 10X.

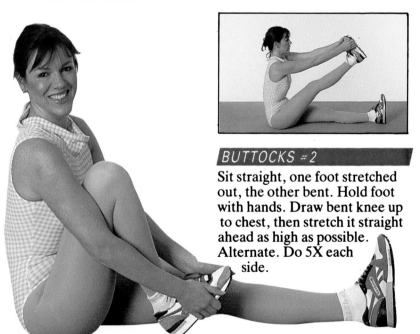

BUTTOCKS ≠2

Sit straight, one foot stretched out, the other bent. Hold foot with hands. Draw bent knee up to chest, then stretch it straight ahead as high as possible. Alternate. Do 5X each side.

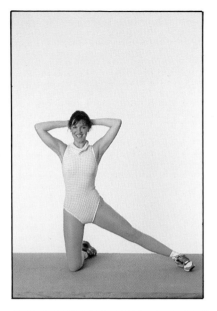

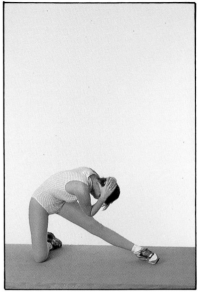

BUTTOCKS #3

Kneel on one knee, other leg stretched to side. Torso straight, and hands clasped behind head.

Twist from waist so elbows touch straight knee. Then return to starting position. Do 5X. Switch sides. Do 5X more.

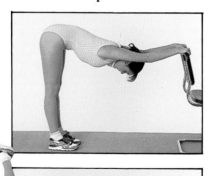

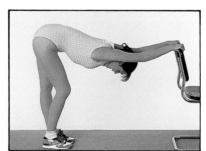

BUTTOCKS #4

Hold back of chair with hands.

Lean body forward and bend one knee.

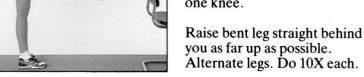

Raise bent leg straight behind you as far up as possible. Alternate legs. Do 10X each.

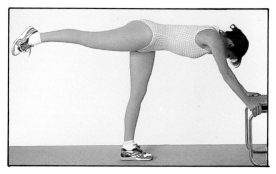

BUTTOCKS #5

Torso is bent, arms are straight and one leg is stretched back, as you hold edge of chair with hands.

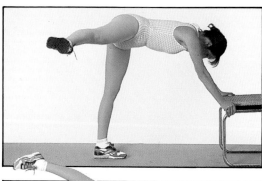

Stretch raised leg to the side.

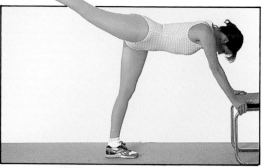

Return to the starting position and alternate legs. Do 10X each.

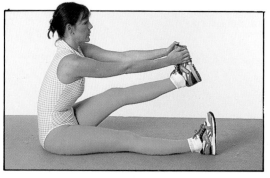

BUTTOCKS #6

Sit on floor with one leg straight, other knee bent, both hands holding foot of bent leg. Stretch bent leg straight out, then up. Hold for count of 5. Alternate legs. Do 10X each.

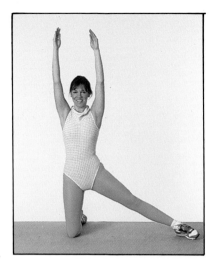

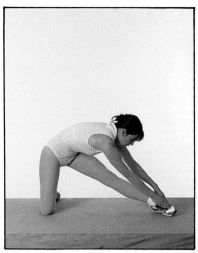

BUTTOCKS #7

With back straight, kneel on one knee and stretch other leg out to side. Hands are raised high.

Twist body so both hands touch toes of outstretched leg. Do 10X. Then switch sides. Do 10X more.

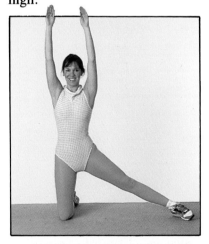

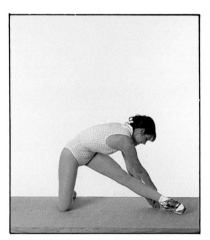

BUTTOCKS #8

Same starting position as above.

This time twist body so both hands touch floor on outer side of straight leg. Then raise body, lift arms high, and try touching floor on outer side of bent knee. Do 10X. Then alternate stance. Do 10X more.

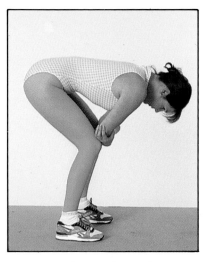
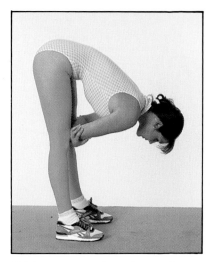

BUTTOCKS #9

Clasp elbows with hands and lean forward, so elbows rest on knees.

Without removing elbows from knees, straighten knees. Slightly bend knees again. Do 10X.

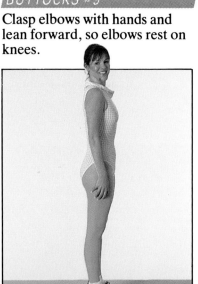
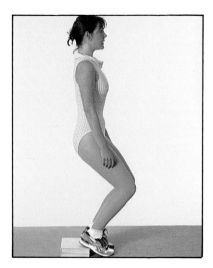

BUTTOCKS #10

Stand with heels on a book or two, toes on floor. Hold on to chair back if necessary.

Bend knees directly over toes, keeping back straight. Return to start. Do 10X. *Note: This exercise should not be done by women who are very overweight, or suffer from knee problems.*

▶ WAIST EXERCISES

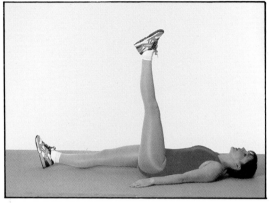

WAIST #1

WAIST #1

Lie on floor with
arms straight out at
sides, palms face
down.
Raise one leg
straight up.

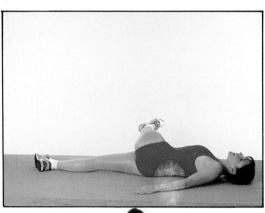

Bring it over body
until side of foot
reaches floor. Raise
leg up again and
lower on opposite
side. Return to start.
Alternate sides. Do
10 repetitions (10X)
each side.

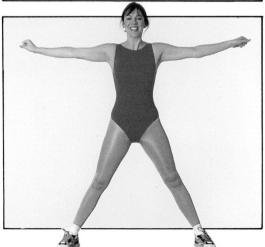

WAIST #2

Feet a giant step
apart, hands with
fists out to sides.

Twist torso so one
hand touches back
of opposite side,
other arm goes up as
high as possible.
Alternate sides. Do
10X each side.

41

WAIST #3

Lie on back, arms to side, legs apart.

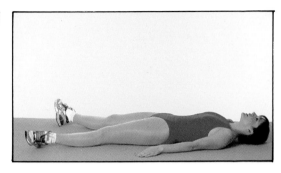

Breathe in, and as you breathe out curl upper body to touch outside left knee. Hold. Repeat on other side. Do 10X.

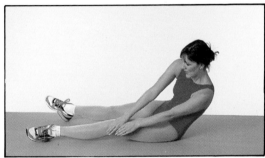

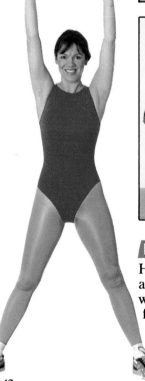

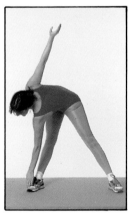

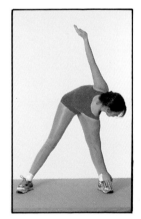

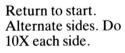

WAIST #4

Hands above head, arms straight, feet wide apart. Gracefully swing from waist until you reach one foot with opposite hand.

Return to start. Alternate sides. Do 10X each side.

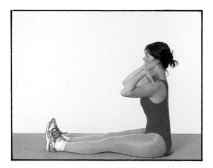

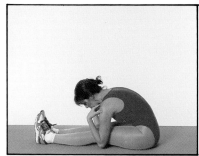

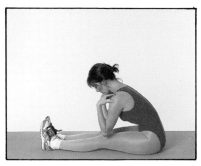

WAIST #5

Sit on floor with feet straight, toes together, hands touching shoulders.
With shoulders level, slowly roll upper body forward so elbows reach knees as close as possible. Slowly uncoil to return to start. Do 10X.

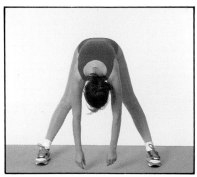

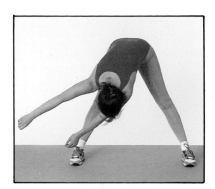

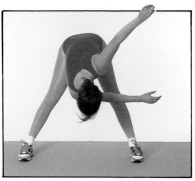

WAIST #6

Bend from standing position with feet wide apart. Let head hang down.

Loosely swing arms from side to side.

Do 25 quick swings.

Stand with one hand behind neck, the other way from body slightly. Feet wide apart.

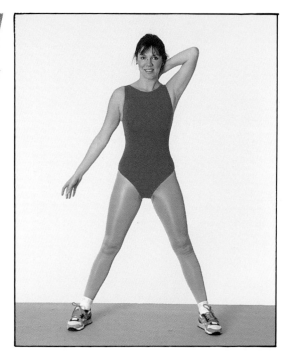

Twist upper body so bent elbow touches opposite knee as straight arm moves up and back. Do 10×. Switch sides. Do 10× more.

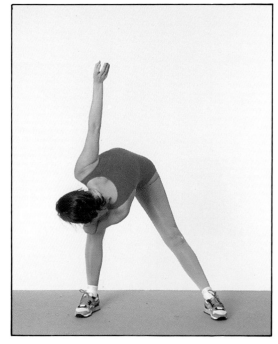

▶ *STOMACH EXERCISES*

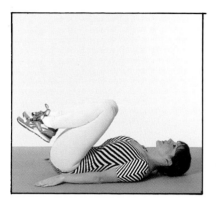

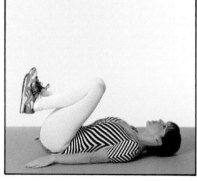

STOMACH #1

Lie on back with knees bent, heels up, toes touching floor. Palms are down at sides. Bring both knees toward chest as much as possible.

Flex feet so toes point up. Hold for count of 5. Return to start. Do 10 repetitions (10X).

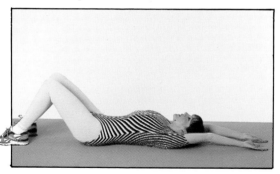

STOMACH #2

Lie on back, knees bent, arms stretched back with palms up.

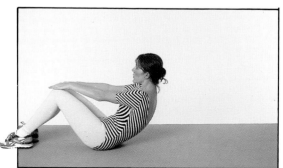

Roll forward into sit-up position, with arms stretched ahead. Hold for count of 5.

Unroll to start. Do 10X.

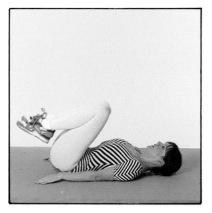

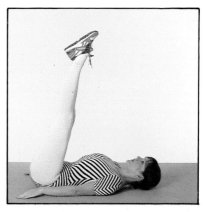

STOMACH #3

On floor, hands at sides, legs straight ahead, with toes pointed forward. Bring both knees in toward chest.

Raise legs up, keeping toes pointed.

Lower to start position. Do 10X.

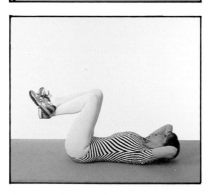

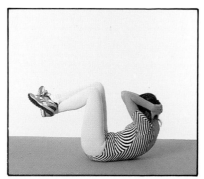

STOMACH #4

On back, hands clasped behind head, feet raised with ankles crossed and knees slightly bent.

Raise torso so elbows reach knees as close as possible. Slowly lower to start. Do 10X.

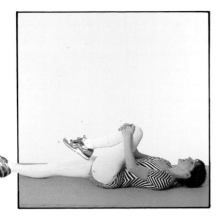

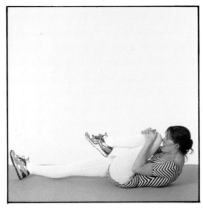

STOMACH #5

Lie on floor with one leg straight. Bend other knee and grasp with both hands.

Raise head. Roll up torso, trying to touch bent knee with nose.

Uncoil to start. Do 5X. Switch sides. Do 5X more.

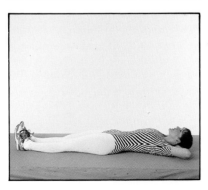

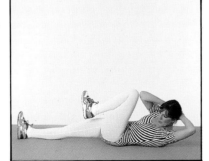

STOMACH #6

On back, hands clasped behind head, legs extended straight ahead.

With head and chest lifted, pull one knee to chest. Touch bent knee with opposite elbow. Return to start. Alternate sides. Do 10X each side.

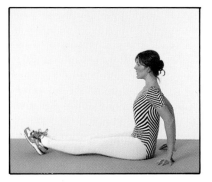

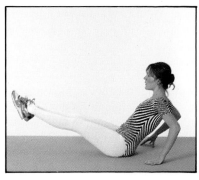

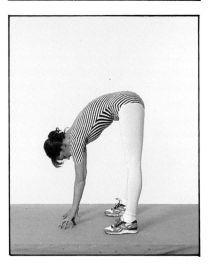

STOMACH #7

Sit on floor; hands behind you.

Raise both legs together.

Lower legs to floor, alternately crossing them. Lift legs up again, repeat. Do 10X.

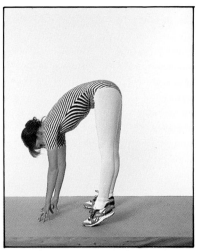

STOMACH #8

Bend down on hands and feet with body lifted, feet apart.

Stand on tiptoe, hold for a few seconds, then lower heels. Do 10X.

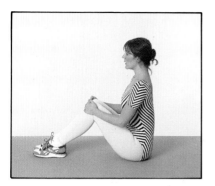

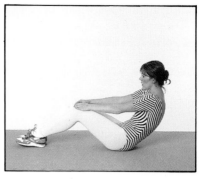

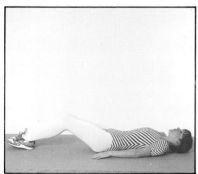

STOMACH #9

Sit on floor with hands clasped around bent knees.

Roll backward to lying position.

Hold for a few seconds, then roll forward to sit up again. Do 10X.

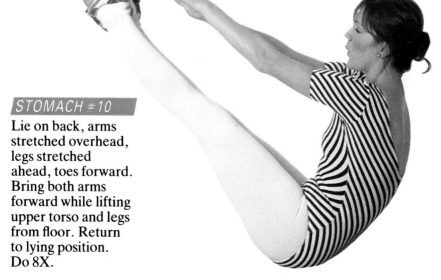

STOMACH #10

Lie on back, arms stretched overhead, legs stretched ahead, toes forward. Bring both arms forward while lifting upper torso and legs from floor. Return to lying position. Do 8X.

▶ COOL-DOWN EXERCISES

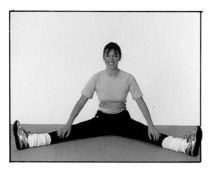

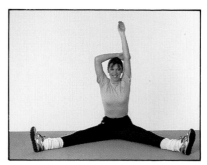

COOL-DOWN #1

Sit with feet wide apart, back
straight, hands on knees.
Bring one arm straight up over
head.
Grasp its elbow with other hand
and pull stretched arm toward
opposite side. Hold for count of
5. Alternate sides. Do 5
repetitions (5X) each side.

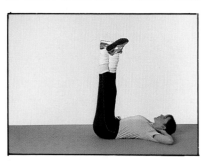

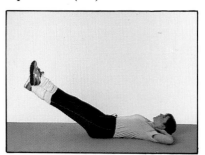

COOL-DOWN #2

Lie on back with legs straight
up, crossed at ankles. Hands
clasped behind head.

Slowly lower legs to floor.

Flex knees in, straighten legs up
again. Do 5X.

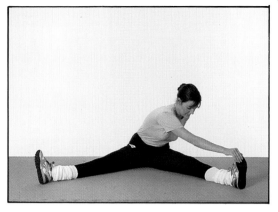

COOL-DOWN #3

Sit on floor with legs wide apart, hands at sides. Twist torso to reach one foot with opposite hand.

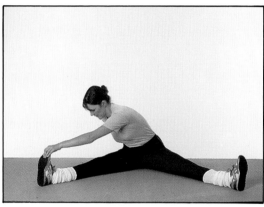

Return to start. Alternate sides. Do 20X.

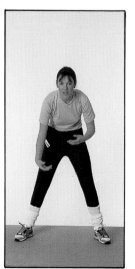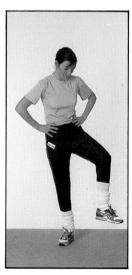

COOL-DOWN #4

Stand with legs moderately apart, arms hanging loosely. Shake both arms.

Then shake alternate legs.

Do 10X arms, 10X each leg.

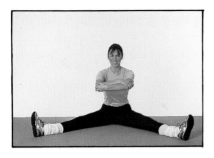 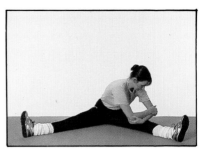

COOL-DOWN #5

Sit with feet wide apart, toes up. Cross arms in front.

Twist forward to touch one knee with elbows.
Return to start. Alternate sides.
Do 10X each side.

COOL-DOWN #6

Lock fingers at waist level while standing with feet moderately apart.
Raise arms straight up, and rotate hands so palms face up. Count to 5. Lower to start. Do 10X.

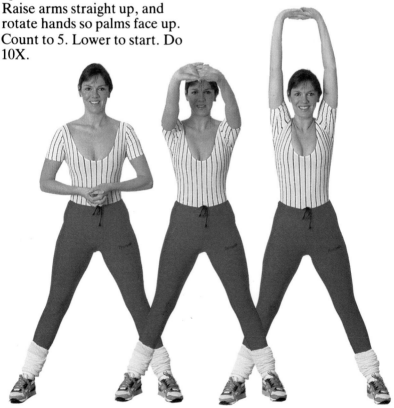

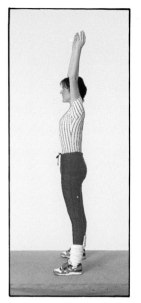 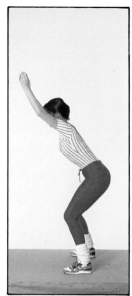 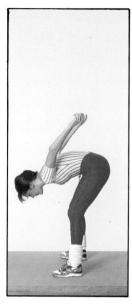

COOL-DOWN #7

Stand straight with hands raised above head.

Lean forward, and bend knees.

Swing elbows behind in a smooth arc. Swing back to start. Do 10X.

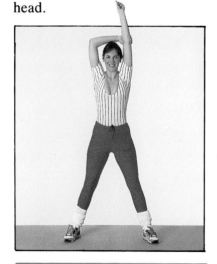 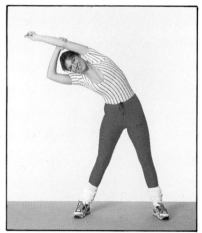

COOL-DOWN #8

Stand with feet wide apart, back straight, one hand straight up, other grasping it by elbow.

Lean body toward bent elbow by pulling straight arm. Count to 5. Return to start. Do 5X each side.

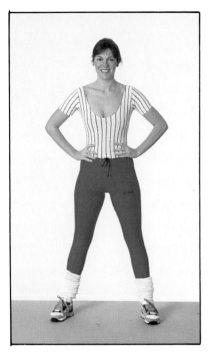

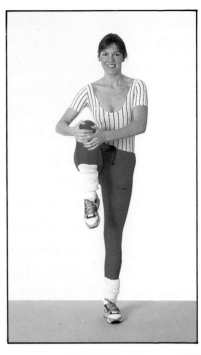

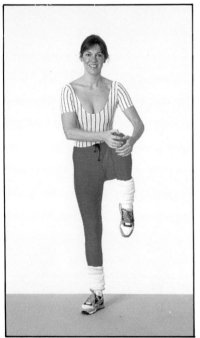

COOL-DOWN #9

Stand with feet slightly apart, elbows bent at waist.

Bring one knee up to chest level. Hold with hands for count of 5.

Alternate sides. Do 10X each side.

▶ *PRENATAL SHAPE-UP*

Women in good physical shape can generally expect fewer complications in pregnancy and delivery, as well as easier labors. Most doctors recommend a mild exercise program for women who are pregnant. Included in this guide are some routines you may find helpful if you are expecting a child. *Please check with your doctor, however, before beginning any of them.*

Other suggestions for improving this joyous time of your life include the following:

● Take it easy. Don't overexert yourself. Enjoy at least one rest period every day.

● When you bend, do so from your knees, not your waist.

● Before going to sleep at night, elevate your legs to increase circulation and counter fatigue. You can do this by placing a pillow beneath your feet.

● If sleep is a problem, try drinking warm milk sweetened with a little honey. A backrub might work nicely, too.

● Help prevent varicose veins by not standing or sitting for too long a period at any one time. Wear loose clothing that isn't restrictive. Support stockings may also be advised.

● Arise slowly in the morning, avoiding erratic movements that may make you feel queasy.

● Choose a firm mattress to sleep on, or use a bed board between your mattress and box spring.

● For immediate relief of leg cramps, flex your toes up toward your knee, or stand without shoes on a cold floor. Leg cramps may indicate you are not getting enough calcium in your diet.

● Develop regular bowel habits. Eating fiber-rich foods helps avoid constipation, as does drinking six to eight glasses of fluid each day.

● If you smoke, now's the time to break the habit. Low birth-weight babies are more common in mothers who are smokers.

● When travelling, choose the most comfortable, least exhausting way. If possible, change your position often on your trip.

● Cut down on your salt intake to help prevent your tissues from retaining fluid, which could result in a serious condition known as edema.

● Watch your weight. While you certainly shouldn't starve yourself, too much weight gain can cause strains on your back and leg muscles, as well as labor complications.

● Expect mood changes. Some days, for no reason, you may feel blue. Normally, such moods will pass.

● Avoid alcohol and caffeine.

▶ *PRENATAL EXERCISES*

Sit with legs crossed in front, arms straight out in front of you.

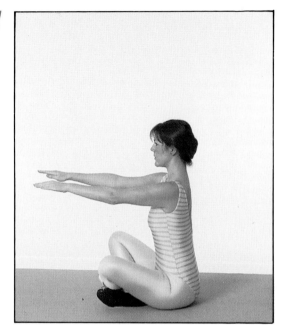

Bring arms over head, fingertips pointing upward. Do 5 repetitions (5X).

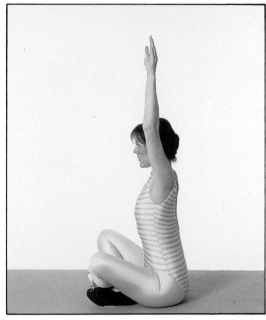

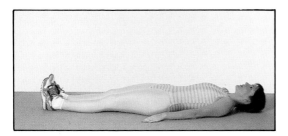

PRENATAL #2

Lie on floor, arms at sides, legs straight ahead.

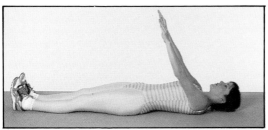

Bring arms back until hands are above head.

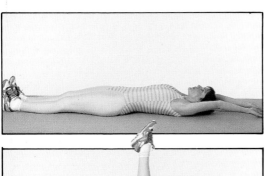

Continue the movement until arms rest behind head. Return to start. Do 5X.

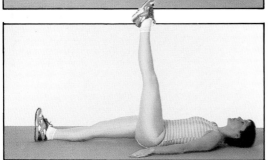

PRENATAL #3

Lie on floor with legs straight ahead. Slowly raise one leg straight up with toes pointed.

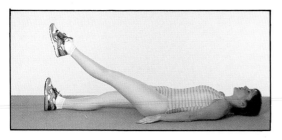

Flex foot. Slowly lower. Do 5X each leg.

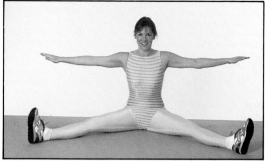

PRENATAL #4

Sit on floor with feet spread out and hands stretched out to sides.

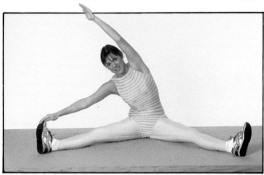

From waist, lean to touch hand to foot on same side, while opposite arm goes up. Alternate sides. Do 5X each side.

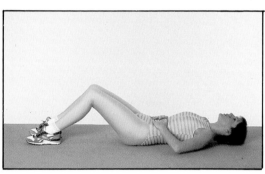

PRENATAL #5

Lie on back, with knees bent.

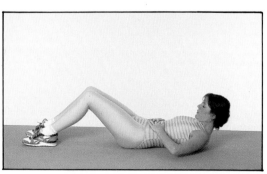

Raise head and try reaching chest with chin. Do not overexert . Do 5X.

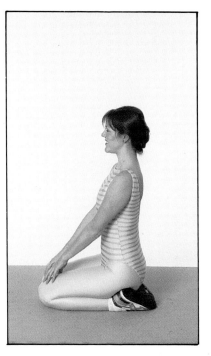
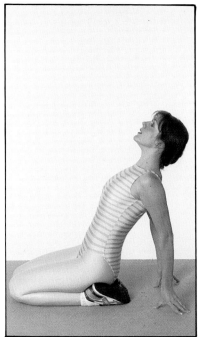

PRENATAL #6

Sit on heels with hands on knees and back straight.

Bring hands to floor behind back.

Arch back, and lower head. Return to start. Do 5X.

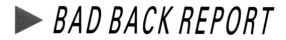

BAD BACK REPORT

In case you haven't guessed it, after the common cold, backaches are the leading cause of employees across the country having to miss work. One estimate reports that Americans lose 10 million work days each year due to backaches. Statistics further show that one out of every three Americans suffers from back problems, especially lower back pain.

Acute back pain is treated with such remedies as bedrest, massage, heat, sleeping on a firmer mattress, a hard board or the floor, and stretching exercises. Recent medical findings indicate that mild back pain goes away in a week or two regardless of whether the sufferer remains in bed or not.

Indications also show that mild backaches can be prevented. This vulnerable area of your body weakens with age. However, you can exercise your lower back muscles to help them keep their youthful elasticity. Exercising also tones up your stomach muscles, which help give your back the support it needs.

Below are some suggestions to keep your back in good working order so you don't miss any time at work . . . or play.

● Practice good posture. Stand straight, sit tall. By doing so, you give your skeleton optimal support, and minimal muscle strain. Slouching and slumping only encourage your spine to weaken.

● Use a firm mattress on your bed, or put a board under a less acceptable mattress.

● Before involving yourself in rigorous back-twisting sports, like tennis or racketball, condition your body with back exercises.

● Bear in mind that such activities as downhill skiing, squash, volleyball and weight training are not advised for people with bad backs.

● Always do warm-up exercises before any workout.

● Don't allow yourself to get overweight. Your balance will be endangered by too much bulk.

● Sleep on your side or back rather than your stomach. Sleeping on your stomach can strain muscles and ligaments in your back. Keep your knees bent when sleeping on your back or side.

● Carry heavy objects in front of you, as near your body as you can. Keep your back straight. If you are forced to lean over backward, the object is too heavy for you to safely carry alone.

● Shift the weight of heavy objects from side to side, rather than favoring one side. Or else, divide up the weight more equally.

● When sitting on the floor without back support, keep a straight back by kneeling, or sitting cross-legged.

● When reading in bed, use a bedboard as well as a pillow to lean back against.
● Choose seats with good back support. Keep both feet on the ground.

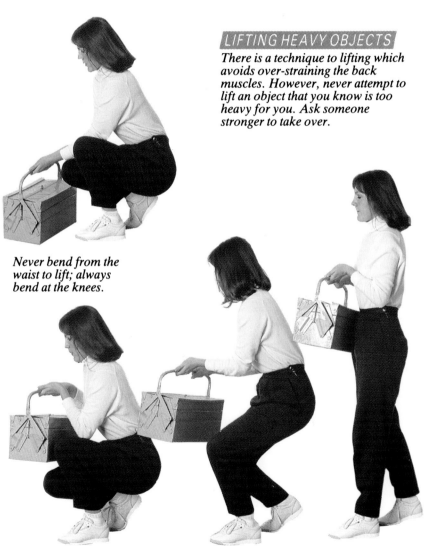

LIFTING HEAVY OBJECTS

There is a technique to lifting which avoids over-straining the back muscles. However, never attempt to lift an object that you know is too heavy for you. Ask someone stronger to take over.

Never bend from the waist to lift; always bend at the knees.

Gradually straighten up, allowing your arms to take the weight rather than your back.

Carry the load in front of you, close to the body, and keep your back straight.

Again, when depositing the load always bend at the knees to bring you down to ground level.

▶ BACK EXERCISES

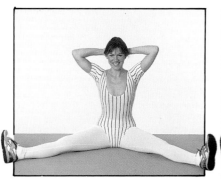

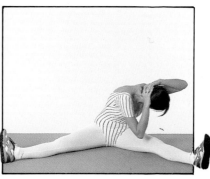

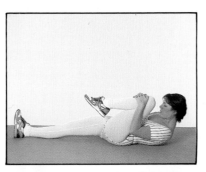

BACK #1

Sit on the floor, with feet wide apart, toes pointing up, and hands clasped behind head.

Twist body so one elbow reaches opposite knee. Return to start.

Alernate sides. Do 10 repetitions (10X) each side.

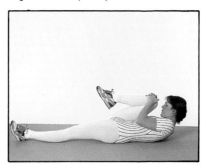

BACK #2

Lie on back with arms at sides, feet straight ahead. Bring one knee in to chest. Grasp with hands and pull upper torso up so nose reaches as near knee as possible. Hold for count of 5.

Alternate knees. Do 5X each side.

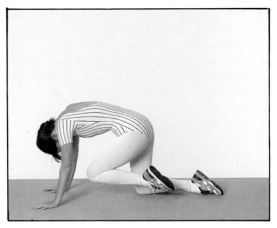

BACK #3

Kneel on hands and knees and draw one knee in toward chest.

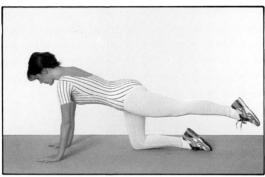

Stretch leg straight back. Return to start.
Alternate legs. Do 5X each side.

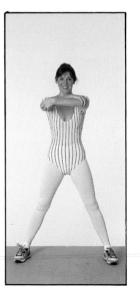 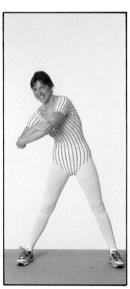

BACK #4

Stand with feet slightly apart, arms folded at eye level.

Move arms, still folded, in circle parallel to floor.

Do 5X toward right, then 5X toward left.

▶ *SLIMMING ON THE SLY*

Busy schedule? You can still sneak in these little exercises to help tone up muscles while you're sitting at your desk, waiting for the bus, even brushing your teeth or riding the elevator. No sense wasting a moment, when fitness is your goal. Note that these little sly slimmers are not meant to substitute for a regular exercise routine. Also, we suggest you *consult a doctor before beginning any exercise regime,* even one that slims you on the sly.

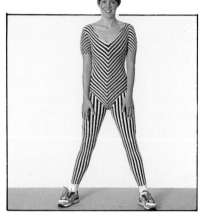

SLY SLIMMER #1

Stand erect, with feet slightly apart, and arms pressed against outsides of thighs.

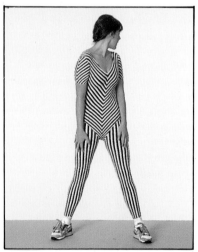

Turn head and upper body to left. Hold for count of 6.

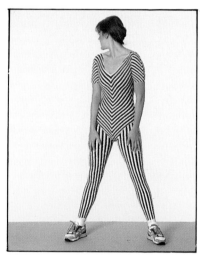

Do 8X each side.

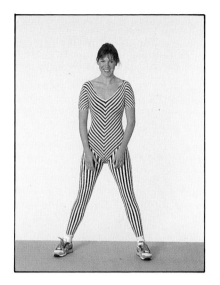

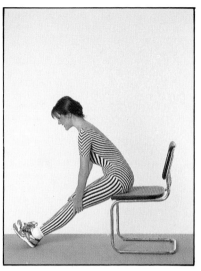

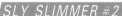

SLY SLIMMER #2

Standing straight, with arms loose at sides, and feet apart, simultaneously tighten abdomen and contract buttocks. Hold for a count of 6. Do 8X.

SLY SLIMMER #3

Sit on a chair, legs straight and hold legs below kneecaps. Push down against legs, and push legs up against hands. Hold for count of 6. Do 8X.

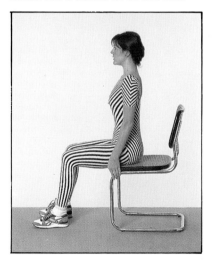

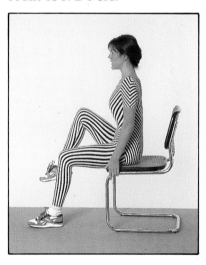

SLY SLIMMER #4

Sitting straight on a chair, grasp

edge of seat with hands. Lift one knee up as far as you can. Do 8X each leg.

WEIGHT TRAINING

Don't mistake weight training for weight lifting. We're not suggesting you become a female equivalent to Mr. America. Those bulging he-man muscles of his come from the male hormone testosterone, which is also present in females, but in much smaller amounts.

Weight training — which requires using barbells or an easy-to-make substitute — is a shortcut to figure firming, thanks to the principle of "progressive resistance." Your muscles, which are in need of toning, are made up of many fibers. The resistance afforded by weights puts more fibers to work than those used in a regular exercise.

The concept is easy to demonstrate. Simply lift up an empty hand. Then lift up one with an object in it. Feel the difference? You've just demonstrated progressive resistance.

Weights can easily be made at home. Raid the kitchen cabinet for them, instead of for a snack.

● A 16-ounce can of fruit or vegetables makes a good one-pound weight.

● For a three-pound weight, try filling a 48-fluid-ounce plastic laundry container (the kind with an easy-to-grasp indented handle) with three pounds of sand or water.

● If you want weights for your feet, fill a double plastic bag with sand equivalent to the desired weight. Secure it closed with rubber bands, and sandwich it between two pieces of material about 12 inches square that have been sewn together on three sides. Now sew up the fourth side, and sew cloth or ribbon ties on all corners to attach the weight to your feet.

Note: Weight-training exercises are not advised for people who suffer from back problems.

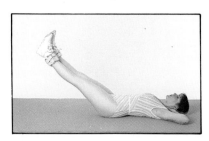

WEIGHT-TRAINING #1

Put ankle weights on. Lie with hands behind head, and raise legs up.

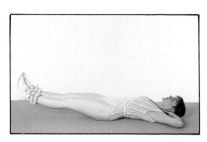

Slowly bring both feet down to floor, then raise them up again. Do 10 repetitions (10X).

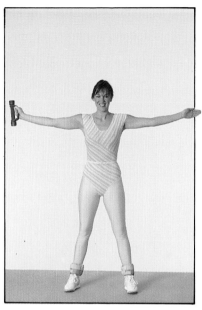

Hold weight in one hand while standing with arms out at shoulder level.

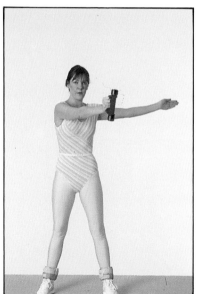

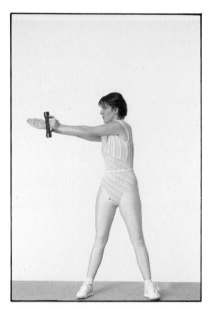

Bring hand with weight across chest to reach other hand. Do 8X.

Then do 8X on opposite side.

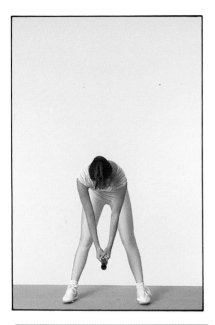

Hold weight with both hands. Stand with legs straight and apart, torso bent forward.

Make circle with arms, bringing weight over head and back down again.

Do 4X toward left side, 4X toward right side.

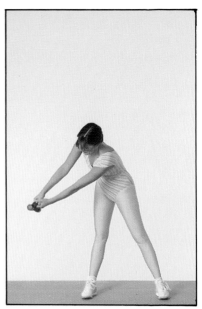

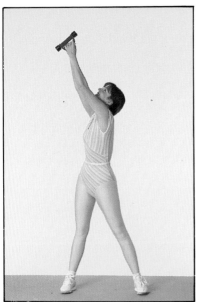

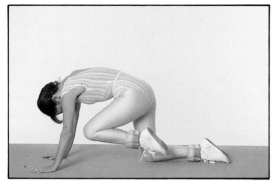

Put ankle weights
on. Kneel on floor
with arms straight,
palms flat on floor,
head face down.
Draw in one knee
until you touch your
chin with it.

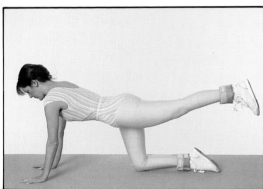

Then stretch it as far
back and up as
possible, while
lifting chin at same
time.

Do 10X each leg.

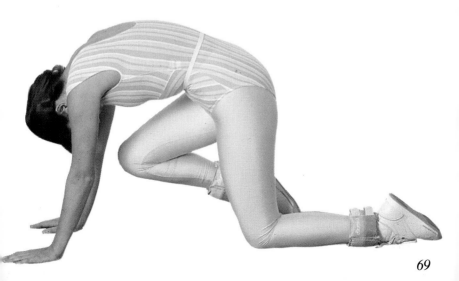

▶ *AEROBICS . . . A HEALTH PHENOMENON*

Over the last few years, aerobics has become far more than just another fitness fad. At last count, approximately 22 million people regularly participated in some kind of aerobic exercise. But how does aerobics differ from regular toning and stretching workouts?

The difference is that shape-up exercises slim you down, but they don't stir up your heart and lungs the way that aerobics do. "Aerobics" refers to a variety of activities that increase the maximum amount of oxygen your body can process in a given amount of time. Your aerobic capacity is the maximum quantity of oxygen your body can process. An effective aerobic exercise has you operating at 70 percent of maximum.

When aerobics are done properly, your entire circulatory and respiratory systems are strengthened. As blood circulates through your body, and your heart pumps with greater efficiency, oxygen is more rapidly sent where it is needed, waste products are more quickly removed, and calories are more effectively burned.

You need to burn off 3,500 calories to get rid of one pound of fat from your body. While half an hour of moderate exercise eliminates 120 to 180 calories, the aerobic activity of jogging at a speed of 5.5 m.p.h. has you burning up approximately 257 calories in the same period of time.

Some of today's most popular aerobic exercises are: brisk walking, jogging, running, swimming, cycling, and aerobic dancing.

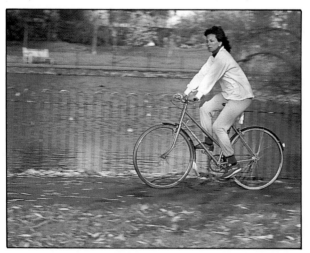

Cycling is both an excellent aerobic exercise and a healthy form of transport for those intermediate distances. If your destination is too far for walking, and too short to merit using the car, rely on pedal-power and enjoy the fresh air and exercise.

MONITOR YOUR PROGRESS

You can monitor your heartbeat and the improvement in your cardiorespiratory system by taking your pulse, which corresponds to your heart rate. For most healthy women, the average at rest pulse (or heart) rate is 70 to 85 beats per minute. As your exercising improves the tone and condition of your cardiorespiratory system, your resting pulse will get lower and lower, until you reach your plateau of peak fitness.

To take your pulse, put one or two fingers of one hand over the radial artery of the other hand. You find this artery by turning your hand palm-up and feeling for the bone on the outer side of your thumb on your wrist. When you locate this bone, move your finger(s) just inside it. Count your pulse for 10 seconds (starting with 0). Then multiply your result by six to obtain your heartbeat per minute.

When you exercise, you want your heart rate to be at 70 percent of its maximum. Estimate your maximum heart rate by subtracting your age from 220 beats per minute. (As you get older, your maximum heart rate decreases.)

You are overexerting your body if your heart rate — or pulse — is over 120 five minutes after your exercising is done.

Monitor yourself at the end of your warm-up period, once or twice during your exercise routine, and five minutes after you are finished cooling down.

Many physical-fitness experts recommend alternating aerobic exercises with toning exercises, so that you put the benefits of both into your schedule.

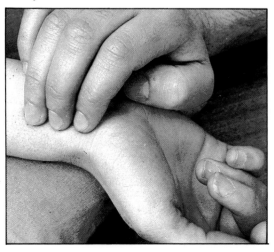

Monitoring your pulse-rate before, during and five minutes after your exercise routine will help you to determine your level of fitness.

▶ *THREE AEROBIC FAVORITES: JOGGING, WALKING, DANCING*

JOGGING

If jogging interests you, don't think you need to enter marathons to reap the benefits of aerobics. You can proceed at your own pace, and still rev up your system, while burning up extra calories.

Some helpful hints for beginner joggers are:

● Start slow, and build up your stamina. Don't expect to be at top performance at once.

● Keep your back straight and head up while running.

● Land heel first with toes pointing forward.

● Never hold your breath while jogging. Breathe deeply, with your mouth open.

● Wear properly-fitted running shoes with good arch supports and firm, cushioned soles. Heavy, soft socks are also suggested in the beginning to guard against shock and blisters.

● Don't let yourself get dehydrated. Drink plenty of fluids, especially on hot, humid days.

● Keep arms slightly away from body, elbows flexed, while running.

● To help prevent tight muscles, warm-up exercises before jogging, and cool-down exercises immediately after, are recommended.

● Allow your body a cooling-off period before taking a hot bath or shower.

● Run on softer surfaces at first to prevent leg injuries.

● Stop running if you feel unusually exhausted or uncomfortable.

Combining exercise with a hobby, such as dance, or with a love of the outdoors, whether walking or jogging, adds purpose to your routine.

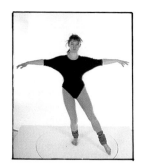
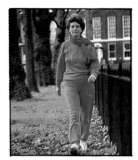

WALKING

Walking is gaining new popularity these days. While it takes longer than jogging to give you the same aerobic benefits, walking also happens to be good all-round exercise. When you walk, you give your whole body — right down to your eye muscles — a workout.

Walking is a great pastime to share with friends, relatives, and neighbors. Set aside half an hour to an hour for a brisk walk after dinner, and you may find it not only offers you a chance to exercise, but also to share fresh air and catch up on friendly chatter.

To benefit from walking, choose shoes with good, thick soles, and a solid heel support. It is also advisable to do five minutes of warm-ups before setting out on your walking adventure.

As with jogging, pace your walking program. Start at a slow pace, on level ground, and set your early goals for short distances at a brisk, yet moderate stride. Keep your movements fluid, rather than bouncy. As your conditioning improves, you'll safely build up both pace and distance.

Your timing is different in walking than jogging. Since you take more steps when you walk than run over the same distance, you use different muscles. And remember that a brisk 45-minute walk during which you tone and strengthen your calves, thighs, ankles, feet, arms, shoulders, abdomen, hips, and buttocks has you burning up 300 calories.

So get into the habit of walking. Walk to work if you can, walk at lunchtime, at coffee breaks, to meetings and appointments. You'll find it's not only a great exercise, but it will also help you get to know your neighborhood a whole lot better.

DANCING

Aerobic dance fever has swept the nation. You see it on TV and read about one class after another popping up in communities everywhere. The rationale is obvious. Aerobic dancing is a fun, sociable activity that's also good for you. What's more, it's available rain or shine, since most classes are held indoors.

Before signing up for an aerobic dance class, ask to watch a session in progress. See if you enjoy how the class is being conducted. Observe the teacher's style and the level of instruction. Then make your choice, and let aerobic dance fever help you become the belle of the ball!

Another choice that is yours today is video classes. If you have a VCR, you might want to explore what exercise tapes are available in your area to rent or buy. Take your pick, and bring the video exercise instructor you like best right into your living room to enjoy in private, or with your friends.

▶ *NUTRIENTS, THE BASIC FOUR + ONE, AND YOU*

Nutrients are needed for basic body well-being. As no one food can give you every nutrient you require, it is vital that you consume a variety of food types in order to obtain the nourishment your body needs. The five basic nutrients are: proteins, carbohydrates, fats, vitamins, and minerals.

The United States Department of Agriculture suggests a basic five group from which they recommend foods to be eaten daily for a balanced, nourishing diet. This expansion from the basic four you probably were taught about as a child is in realistic appraisal of American diets in the 1980s. However, people who want to reduce are recommended to cut portions of the fifth group (fats, sweets and alcohol) first, as this is the group that contains the least amount and variety of nutrients. Then, if excess weight is still a problem, USDA nutritionists suggest reducing the size of portions in the other four groups. These are the groups and their recommended servings for average adults:

FRUIT AND VEGETABLES

Four servings a day; one should be a source rich in Vitamin C such as oranges. Also recommended for frequent consumption are Vitamin A vegetables such as carrots. Fruits and vegetables provide carbohydrates, minerals, and vitamins, as well as fiber. They are also low in calories.

BREADS AND CEREALS

Four servings a day, preferably whole-grained products that naturally contain fiber, an important element in your diet. (Fortified or enriched products do not provide this.) Included in this group are pasta, rice, cereal and baked goods, which provide carbohydrates, proteins, minerals, and vitamins.

MILK AND CHEESE

Includes yogurt and ice cream, and provides protein, calcium, and riboflavin. If fortified, milk contains Vitamin D as well. Recommended servings for adults vary: in general, however, adults should have two servings: pregnant women three servings; nursing mothers four servings.

MEAT, POULTRY, FISH, AND BEANS

Two servings daily are recommended to provide protein, vitamins, and minerals. A serving equals two to three ounces of lean, cooked meat, poultry or fish without bone. A serving of one egg equals one ounce of meat. So, too, do ½ to ¾ cups of nuts, sesame seeds, or sunflower seeds.

ALCOHOL, FATS, AND SWEETS

Moderation is the key. This is the first group to cut down on when losing weight. It includes mayonnaise, salad oils, margarine, butter, cream, soft drinks, candy, deep-fried foods, and all alcoholic drinks.

If you want to combine muscle toning with permanent weight loss, nutritionists suggest you follow a standard 1,200-calorie daily food allowance, while at the same time changing your pattern of eating for life.

To understand the principle behind the suggested daily calorie allowance, you need to know some simple facts about calories; your friend or enemy, depending on how you use them.

Basically, calories are a unit of measure for the amount of energy — or heat — you get from food. This energy is either used immediately to perform muscular work or routine body functions, or else it is stored in reserve as fat. If this fat reserve is not used up, it gets larger and larger, and you need to lose weight.

Each time you ring up 3,500 calories of reserved energy in your fat vault, you become a pound heavier. Likewise, whenever you get rid of 3,500 calories, you become a pound lighter.

To find out the amount of calories required to maintain your ideal weight, multiply that figure (in pounds) by 12. How many calories are you currently taking in? You'll find that number by multiplying your present weight by 12.

(To be even more accurate, you will want to make an age adjustment. For every year after age 25, reduce your caloric input by 10 calories. Or else, increase your activity.)

The dieter's standard 1,200-calorie daily food plan, combined with your exercise regime, will allow you a safe weight loss of one to two pounds per week. When you want to lose 10 or more pounds, shedding only one or two weekly may seem a slow, hard grind. But remember this is the beginning of a weight loss that will be permanent, healthy, and well worth the effort.

▶ *HEALTHY FOOD HABITS*

Food habits develop for most of us in childhood. Develop new habits now, and your "eating lifestyle" can be restructured so that weight ceases to be a problem, and good health will be a constant for you. Here are some good ways to help you reach the goal of a healthier eating pattern.

● Snack on foods that are non-fattening. Keep raw vegetables handy to satisfy between-meal food cravings. Nibble-size portions of vegetables such as broccoli, carrots, celery, mushrooms, and string beans can keep your tummy satisfied as well as slim. You can enjoy most vegetables without worrying about weight gain.

● Satisfy your thirst with water. And for an elegant noncaloric thirst quencher, try mineral water with a twist of lemon or lime. Six to eight glasses of fluid a day are recommended to flush your system and keep you feeling pleasantly full.

● Shop on a full stomach. This will prevent "the hungries" from making you pile up your shopping cart with more food than you need. While you're at it, stroll right past the candy and cookie aisles in the supermarket. Spend more time in the fresh produce section, and stock up on nutrient-rich edibles.

● Eat slowly. Enjoy each forkful that goes into your mouth. Pause during meals. When you've finished an average portion, take a breather, even if you're still hungry. Give your brain the time it requires to get the message that you're full.

● Regulate portions at the table. Instead of serving family style, dole out what you, and everyone else, gets at dinnertime. This is a precaution against anyone overindulging.

● Include bulk (fiber) in your diet. Bulk will help your system run more effectively. Such bulk comes from salad fixings, as well as from fruits, vegetables, and whole-grain breads.

● Check your weight once a week, with the same amount of clothes on, at the same time of day, (early morning preferred), and on the same scale. Most women find daily weigh-ins too frustrating, since fluctuations in day-to-day water retention for women gives inaccurate readings.

● Stress and food make poor companions. Don't eat when you're upset, since you may bloat yourself under pressure.

● Don't skip meals. The danger of doing so is that it will increase your desire to snack. Instead, stick to the traditional three meals a day.

● A snapshot of the figure you're determined to change fastened to your refrigerator can work wonders toward keeping you from giving in to snack attacks.

▶ *THE DANGERS OF DIETS*

When people think about losing weight, diets immediately come to mind. What diet to try? At last count, there were some 4,000 different kinds reported. Chances are, you've tried your fair share of them. But before starting another, consider that many nutrition experts advise against what have come to be known as "fad diets," eating plans that promise huge weight losses in short periods of time. Some are dangerous — like the heralded liquid diet of a few years back that wound up causing at least 15 deaths.

Over the last few years there've been milk and banana diets, hamburger diets, spaghetti diets, and even lollipop diets. You've probably heard about many diets whose inventors have made fortunes with best-selling books. People do lose weight on such diets, if they stick to them.

But the proof of the pudding — non-fattening or otherwise — is whether the weight stays off. Fad or crash diets often have you losing weight while you're on them, only to gain it back again when you stop in what is known as the "yo-yo" syndrome of weight loss and gain. This endangers the balance of your system, and can result in illness, rather than better health.

Fad diets can also be dangerous. They limit the nutrients your system needs to operate efficiently. Most nutritionists agree that the best way to lose weight and keep it off permanently is with a low-calorie, well-balanced diet that gradually gets incorporated into your total lifestyle.

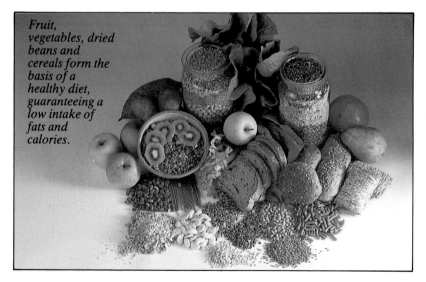

Fruit, vegetables, dried beans and cereals form the basis of a healthy diet, guaranteeing a low intake of fats and calories.

▶ THE WORST DIETARY OFFENDERS

Be especially cautioned against fat, sodium, and sugar.

FAT

Eating too much fat can not only increase your weight, but can also seriously endanger your health. Build-ups of fats and cholesterol in the coronary arteries that supply the heart muscle with the vital blood it needs can result in a condition called arteriosclerosis. In time, this condition can cause one of the major arteries to be blocked, resulting in chest pain, a heart attack, stroke or sudden death. If health is a concern, then limiting your fat intake — and that of your family — should be taken seriously.

The National Academy of Sciences has also reported evidence linking some common cancers to excess fat in diets. What can be done? The average American gets approximately 40 percent of her calories from fat. Many experts recommend reducing this to about 30 percent. Fats are naturally present in foods, are added in processing and cooking, and are added at the table. Here are some tips to reduce fat intake:

● Choose lean cuts of meat and poultry. Trim off the skin and visible fat.

● Whenever possible, avoid processed foods such as frankfurters, sausage, and salami. They have a higher fat content than lean meats.

● Increase your intake of fish, which is naturally low in fat. When choosing canned fish, look for water packs instead of oil.

● Cut down on fats in cooking. Instead of frying foods, bake or broil them. Also try stir frying, which uses only a small amount of oil and cooks foods quickly over a high flame. Or use a non-stick pan. It requires no oil.

● Drain meats after cooking.

● At the table, limit the amount of butter or margarine used on bread. Substitute lemon juice as a vegetable enhancer.

● Use less oil in salad dressings. If creamy dressings are your downfall, try them with a plain yogurt base.

SODIUM

Sodium makes up 40 percent of salt. Most Americans use too much sodium in their diets. While sodium is required in small amounts for proper body functioning, it can also become a major health hazard for people with above-normal blood pressure. High blood pressure can result in damage to your organs, especially your brain, heart, and kidneys.

The amount of salt in our diet can be controlled. But beware that sodium comes from other sources than salt. It can also be found in baking powder, baking soda, and monosodium glutamate. To lower your sodium intake, here are some helpful guidelines:

● The National Research Council of the National Academy of Sciences indicates that 1,100 to 3,300 milligrams of sodium a day are "safe and adequate" for adults. Read the package labels to see what your servings will reap. Expect convenience and processed foods to have higher sodium contents than natural, fresh foods.

● When snacking, choose unsalted nuts and popcorn, rather than the salted variety of either, and avoid potato chips and other salted snack foods altogether.

● Reduce the amount of salt you use in cooking. Substitute other flavorings. Pepper, garlic, basil, and oregano, to name just a few, can pep up foods without adding sodium. Wine and fruit juices can also enhance taste when cooking. Also, totally bar the salt shaker from the dinner table.

SUGAR

Sucrose, the refined, sweet white granules found in sugar bowls on American tables is just one kind of sugar. Other caloric sweeteners such as corn syrup are used in food manufacturing. While honey and molasses are two sweeteners that contain traces of some vitamins and minerals, their nutrient contribution to a diet is insignificant, and the nutrient content of other sugars is even less. Sugar intake is also the major culprit in tooth decay. Here are some ways to reduce sugar intake:

● Check labels carefully. Learn to identify the terms that mean sugar is present. If sugar, sucrose, glucose, maltose, dextrose, lactose, fructose or syrups appear as one of the first three ingredients on a label, you can be sure that there are large amounts of sugar in the product.

● When you crave a sweet treat, choose fruits. They have a natural sugar content, as well as a variety of nutrients.

● When baking, reduce the amount of sugar called for in a recipe. Do this gradually to achieve a product you and your family find worthy of compliments. Often less sweet variations taste just fine, if not better, than the original recipe.

● Cut down on sugary soft drinks. A 12-ounce container of cola contains some nine teaspoons of sugar.

▶ EATING OUT WITHOUT GUILT

Today's busy woman is apt to eat out a great deal, in restaurants or at social engagements rich in culinary temptations. True, an occasional dietary splurge won't destroy a figure, or a diet. But when eating out is a regular routine, it helps to have some guidelines to make sure eating away from home doesn't become an ongoing excuse for slipping into old patterns of weight gain.

RESTAURANT DINING

When you're dining in restaurants, here are some tips you'll find useful to keep in mind:

● First things first. If possible, choose a restaurant that you're sure will have dishes both healthy and filling. Chinese food offers you more choices than Mexican. An all-American cuisine offers more choices than an Italian one. Many restaurants display their menus in their windows, so you can study them before going inside.

● In a fast-food restaurant, substitute a salad for French fries. If the eatery has a salad bar, build your meal around it. Go for the smallest portion of meat in a hamburger restaurant, and fill up on salad instead. (But avoid chickpeas. They have the same amount of calories per serving as a single-dip sundae. Also, keep your salad dressing down to one teaspoon.) On sandwiches avoid mayonnaise and tartar sauce.

● Ask that any gravies and salad dressings be served on the side, so you can regulate the quantity that you're getting. Then use either sparsely. You'll discover that a little can go a long way.

● Try sticking to plain water if possible. If an alcoholic beverage seems appropriate, request dry white wine — one of the lowest-calorie alcoholic beverages you can find.

● Order food that is broiled, roasted, or poached, rather than breaded, fried, or sautéed. Don't be embarrassed to ask your food server how dishes are prepared, and then request yours made to order. Let your health overcome any hesitation you have to assert your desires.

● If a restaurant is known to serve large portions, ask for less. That way you won't have to rely on your willpower. There will be nothing to tempt you to overindulge. Otherwise, get in the habit of asking for a doggie bag. You don't have to eat everything on your plate. You're not a kid anymore.

● Instead of rich desserts, look for fruit on the menu. If not listed under desserts, check under appetizers, where you may find a melon or fruit cup that will finish off your meal with the perfect touch.

DINING WITH FRIENDS

When eating out means going to someone's house for dinner, here are some simple suggestions to keep you sociable, yet right on target with your weight watching:

● Enjoy a low-calorie snack before leaving home, so you won't be famished when dinner is served. Some plain yogurt, an apple, or a cup of clear bouillon will help.

● If hors d'oeuvres are served, try not to sit close to them. You don't need the temptation. And avoid addictive drink companions like salted nuts, potato chips, and pretzels. One is never enough.

● Buffet style? Stick to the salads, cold cuts, and raw fruits and vegetables, rather than the hot dishes, which are likely to be swimming in rich sauces.

● Compromise your taste buds. If a dish looks delicious, allow yourself a taste, but no more. That way you won't feel deprived, nor will you go overboard. Practice discipline.

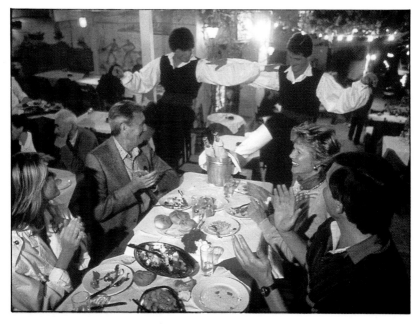

Dining out with friends is a pleasurable experience, but should not be an excuse for over-indulging in the fattening foods you have been resisting in your normal daily diet.

▶ *POSTURE POINTERS*

Many beauty experts call posture the secret key to health and beauty. Good posture gives you a bearing that signals to others that you are someone with both good health and confidence. But standing up straight does far more than make an all-important good first impression on others.

Good posture can relieve muscular tension and help you feel as good as you look. However, this finely tuned "balancing act" requires firm, well-developed hip, buttock, abdomen, and thigh muscles, as well as a strong diaphragm. Is it worth developing? You bet! When your body is properly aligned, with your head held high, your neck and shoulders relaxed, your abdomen flat, you've got on a natural corset.

Still more good news.

Since your muscles won't need to do extra work to compensate for your body's uneven alignment, you'll find yourself peppier as well as more poised.

The best way to check out your own posture is to take a good, honest look at yourself in the mirror. Don't let your posture flaws get you down. The first step toward improvement — and most people can use some — is to consciously face your flaws and consciously begin eliminating them.

Good postural balance is yours if your back is straight, your hips even, your shoulders level, and your head right above your shoulders. Like exercise, good posture is a habit you develop with time, practice, and perseverance.

POSTURE TIPS

To increase your personal poise, and make sure that important first impression is a good one every time, here are some posture secrets worth incorporating into your daily life:

● When sitting down, keep your upper torso straight, tuck your buttocks under, and with your knees slightly bent, gracefully slide into a seated position.

● While seated, keep your back and shoulders straight, abdomen tucked in, and chest out. Keep knees and feet close together on the floor. If you must cross your legs, do so at the ankles, not the knees.

● When rising from your seat, put one foot in front of the other. Then, with your back erect, lean forward from your hips, and gracefully stand up.

● Walk with your movements coming from your hips, while your buttocks and abdomen are tucked in. Hold your head high, and your shoulders back. Consciously avoid swinging your arms or hips.

Remember that even if your figure's svelte, if your posture's not up to par, you won't convey that air of graceful self-confidence you want. So, keep your posture in mind until it becomes second nature to always walk and sit in style and beauty.

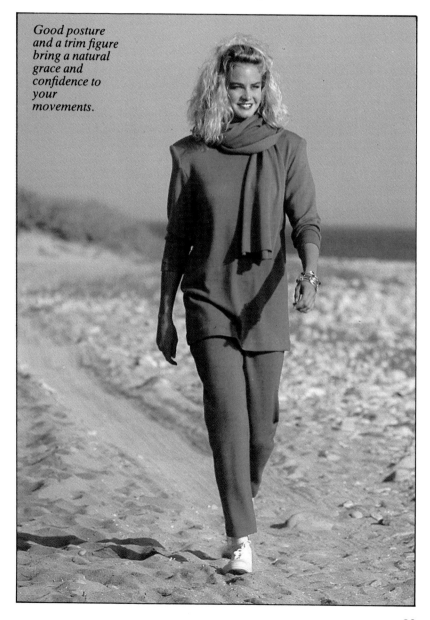

Good posture and a trim figure bring a natural grace and confidence to your movements.

▶ *BREATHING FOR FITNESS*

A deep breath. It's one of the most relaxing, invigorating things we can enjoy. With each inhalation, we draw fresh energy into our bodies. With each exhalation, we banish tiredness.

Yet many people don't breathe properly. Like so many other things we take for granted in life, bad breathing is a habit. Two of the most frequent breathing faults are breathing through the mouth (unlike the nose, it has no filter device, which means it lets impurities like dust and soot enter your system), and drawing in air with the chest rather than the diaphragm.

Rhythmic abdominal breathing helps your body run effectively. When you breathe deeply, you take in larger quantities of oxygen as you inhale and eliminate greater amounts of air you've used up

Yoga is a form of exercise that teaches you the techniques of relaxation, benefiting you both physically and mentally.
Take time out from your busy, hectic schedule and find some space for peace and solitude. Close the door to interruptions, and sit in a comfortable position; ideally cross-legged with back straight and elbows

resting on knees. Close your eyes and take deep, measured breaths from the abdomen. Complete the exercise by letting your head fall forwards for a few minutes. Just five minutes will leave you feeling both relaxed and refreshed and will help you face the rest of the day with added zest.

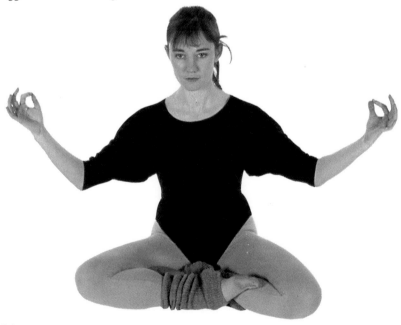

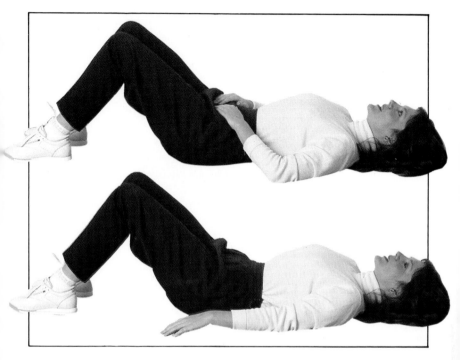

Here is an exercise to help you practice deep abdominal breathing: Lie on your back and bend your knees until your feet rest flat on the floor. Consciously relax all your muscles, from head to toe. Place your hands on your stomach to feel your abdomen move. Then inhale slowly, expanding your abdomen as much as possible without moving your chest. Hold for a count of five. Contract your stomach as much as possible and exhale slowly. Rest for a count of five and repeat five times.

as you exhale. Your circulation and recharging mechanisms are improved.

Breathing deeply is an exercise in itself. You can do it wherever you are. Simply breathe in deeply — being sure to inhale through your nose. Then exhale deeply through your mouth. (Visualize yourself smelling a rose on the inhalation, and blowing out a candle on the exhalation.)

When people first start to exercise, it is not uncommon for them to hold their breath, as if they thought doing so would increase their strength. Instead, it could lead to a phenomenon known as the Valsalva effect, which in effect prevents blood from properly returning to the heart. To avoid such a plight, remember when exercising to exhale on every exertion, and inhale on every return.

Breathing correctly puts to work as many as 17 breathing muscles in your neck, shoulders, and chest.

▶ *COMMON QUESTIONS ABOUT EXERCISE AND DIET*

ARE SAUNAS A GOOD WAY TO LOSE WEIGHT?

While saunas, like steam rooms and hot tubs, may make you feel good, they're not recommended for losing weight. You are sweating away water in them, not fat, and the water loss will most likely be compensated for by the liquids you'll guzzle afterward. Such treatments can also be dangerous. People with hardening of the arteries, heart problems, or excessive thyroid activity are advised to avoid treatments that use heat. Also, heatstroke can result from going directly from strenuous exercise to a sauna, or even a hot shower.

While we're at it, rubber or plastic suits used to induce sweat while exercising are also on the not-recommended list. Such extra clothing prevents heat produced during exercise from escaping the body. This places a greater strain on the heart regulatory mechanism. In brief, what seem like shortcuts to slimming down can be detrimental to your health, instead.

ARE VITAMIN SUPPLEMENTS NECESSARY? IF SO, SHOULD I CHOOSE NATURAL VITAMINS?

Most women don't need vitamin supplements, since a balanced diet will provide the average woman with all the vitamins required. However, doctors may recommend a vitamin or mineral supplement for some women, including: dieters eating less than 1,600 calories a day for an extended period of time, pregnant and nursing women, sufferers from chronic intestinal diseases that affect vitamin and mineral absorption, frequent imbibers of alcohol, patients on long-term medication affecting their nutritional needs, and total vegetarians who digest no animal foods, dairy products or eggs. Consult your doctor to find out if you should be taking a daily supplement.

Since there is no chemical difference between "natural" vitamins and those that are man-made, most doctors agree that it makes no difference to your body whether you take a natural or synthetic supplement.

CAN BREAST SIZE BE CHANGED BY EXERCISE?

There are no bones in the breast. Besides the mammary glands and the nipple (a muscular organ) the breast is primarily connective tissue cushioned by a fatty layer. The pectoral muscles, located on the sides and center of your chest, underlying your breasts, support the breast. The health and elasticity of your pectoral muscles help determine your breast shape, and firmness. Breast size cannot be altered by exercise, since glands and fatty tissue, not muscle, are responsible for size. However, pectorals are a kind of bra. By developing these important muscles, you can uplift a small bosom so that it appears larger. And diet plus exercise aid women with oversized breasts.

MIGHT I BE DESTINED TO BE FAT?

You might be destined to have a harder than average time of losing weight. Studies at Rockefeller University in New York City reveal that overeating in infancy and childhood can increase the number of fat cells in our body. Although diet and exercise can empty these cells of their fat content, they stick around throughout our lives, waiting to be replenished by extra calories.

Scientists have also found body chemicals that regulate how much weight we gain and lose from our caloric intake. An enzyme called lipoprotein lipase (LPL) seems to snatch fatty substances from the blood and store them in fat cells. If recent studies are correct, many chronically overweight people have more LPL in their systems than thinner people do. Another recent study indicates that overweight people may have lower-than-normal levels of APT-ase, an enzyme in red blood cells that governs 20 to 40 percent of the body's heat and energy production. Calories that would normally be used up as heat are converted into fat for these people.

But the good news is that such conditions can be conquered. If you have serious trouble losing weight, even though you really try, your best bet is to check with a doctor.

HOW DO I FIGHT CELLULITE?

In 1973 a new word was introduced to America by a Frenchwoman named Madame Ronsard. The word was "cellulite." It refers to what she considered a "special" fat unique to women, which appears as ripples primarily on the hips and buttocks. The word started an international debate, with some arguing that cellulite exists, and others in the medical community vehement that there is no such specialized fat. But call them what you will, those pock-marked areas of your body known as "cellulite zones" are the result of fat and lack of muscle tone. To eliminate them, your wisest action is to combine adequate exercise with a diet that is nutritionally sound.

HOW DO SATURATED FATS DIFFER FROM POLYUNSATURATED FATS?

Saturated fats are usually of animal origin; for example, butter, dairy products, and the fat found in meats. These fats tend to elevate the cholesterol level in your blood. Saturated fats contain as much hydrogen as they possibly can hold.

In contrast, polyunsaturated fats are usually of vegetable origin; for example, corn, safflower, and soybean oil. They contain less hydrogen and tend to lower the blood's cholesterol level.

There is a third type of fat, known as monounsaturated, that has no effect on blood cholesterol level. Peanut oil and olive oil are two monounsaturated fats. Monounsaturated or polyunsaturated fat products should be used in preference to saturated ones by those concerned about cholesterol.

HOW DOES MARGARINE DIFFER FROM BUTTER?

Butter is derived from animal sources. Margarine comes from vegetable sources. The source of their fat is thus different, but the calories each contains are the same.

ARE NON-DAIRY CREAMERS BETTER THAN CREAM IN MY COFFEE?

Most non-dairy creamers come from coconut oil, which is a saturated fat. If you want to lower your saturated fat intake, neither cream nor non-dairy creamers are advised.

HOW SHOULD I DETERMINE WHAT I SHOULD WEIGH?

Height and weight charts with "average" weights for women of a given height and frame do exist. However, frame size is often vague, and not everyone who is the same height should weigh the same.

A popular method in use today allows 100 pounds for the first five feet and five pounds per inch over five feet. You are also asked to add five pounds additional for a medium frame, and 10 pounds extra for a large frame.

Another standard some use is that you weigh throughout your life the weight that was desirable for you in your mid-twenties.

Your ideal weight is perhaps best determined by a combination of weight charts and common sense about how you feel. Most people can "feel" what weight is right for them, no matter what standard charts may say, and it is wiser to trust your instinct and your mirror in such cases.

WILL IDEAL WEIGHT CHARTS TELL ME HOW FAT I AM?

No. You can be fatter than you think. It's an excess of fat on the inside of your body that we're referring to; fat that can compress your organs, such as the heart, lungs, kidneys, and liver. An average woman should have 20 to 27 percent fat as a percentage of her total weight. A swimming pool is the public's counterpart to the more scientific underwater immersion test. With over 25 percent body fat, you float with ease. You float while breathing shallowly with 22 to 23 percent fat. With 15 percent fat, you sink slowly.

A simple at-home procedure to determine your percentage of body fat is the "pinch test". Grab a fold of skin on either side of your abdomen, hips or upper arms. While holding the fold between thumb and forefinger, measure its width with a tape measure. If it measures over ¾ inch, you're over-fat.

Remember that ideal weight charts don't really tell whether you're too fat. You could slip into a perfect size-eight dress, yet poor muscle tone and fat could have you sagging and unhealthy, rather than stunning and in tip-top condition.

DESIRABLE WEIGHTS FOR WOMEN AGED 25 AND OVER
(in pounds, in indoor clothing)

Height		Small frame	Medium frame	Large frame
Feet	Inches			
4	10	92– 98	96–107	104–119
4	11	94–101	98–110	106–122
5	0	96–104	101–113	109–125
5	1	99–107	104–116	112–128
5	2	102–110	107–119	115–131
5	3	105–113	110–122	118–134
5	4	108–116	113–126	121–138
5	5	111–119	116–130	125–142
5	6	114–123	120–135	129–146
5	7	118–127	124–139	133–150
5	8	122–131	128–143	137–154
5	9	126–135	132–147	141–158
5	10	130–140	136–151	145–163
5	11	134–144	140–155	149–168
6	0	138–148	144–159	153–173

Source: U.S. Public Health Service

TWO-WEEK PROGRESS REPORT

Keep tabs on your improved fitness, diligently record your progress every two weeks. Rate your general mental outlook and energy level on a scale of 1 to 10 with 10 being maximum. And feel proud! Look at the strides you've made!

DATE						
WEIGHT						
MEASUREMENTS						
Left Ankle						
Right Ankle						
Left Calf						
Right Calf						
Left Knee						
Right Knee						
Left Thigh						
Right Thigh						
Left Hip						
Right Hip						
Waist						
Midriff						
Bust						
Left Arm						
Right Arm						
GENERAL WELL-BEING						
Mental Outlook						
Energy Level						

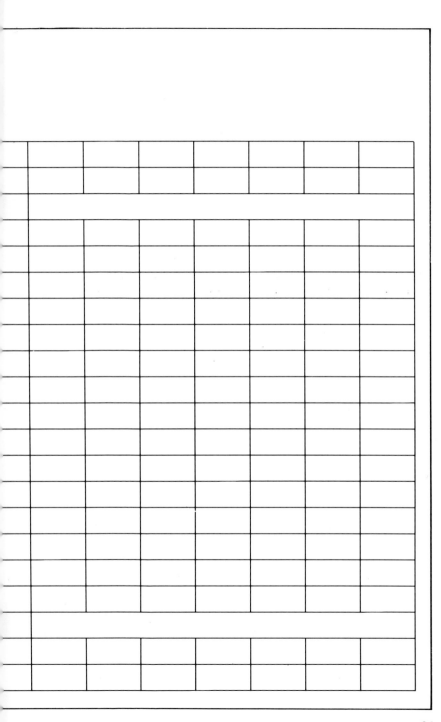

TWO-WEEK PROGRESS REPORT

Keep tabs on your improved fitness, diligently record your progress every two weeks. Rate your general mental outlook and energy level on a scale of 1 to 10 with 10 being maximum. And feel proud! Look at the strides you've made!

DATE						
WEIGHT						
MEASUREMENTS						
Left Ankle						
Right Ankle						
Left Calf						
Right Calf						
Left Knee						
Right Knee						
Left Thigh						
Right Thigh						
Left Hip						
Right Hip						
Waist						
Midriff						
Bust						
Left Arm						
Right Arm						
GENERAL WELL-BEING						
Mental Outlook						
Energy Level						

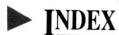 **INDEX**

Page numbers in *italic* refer to the illustrations and captions

Aerobics, 70
dancing, *72*, 73
jogging, *7, 72*
walking, *72*, 73
Alcohol:
pregnant women, 55
recommended
servings, 75
Arms:
swinging, 13, 14
upper, 31-5

B

Back exercises, 60, 62-3
Back problems, 60-1
carrying heavy objects, 60
lifting heavy objects, 61, *61*
mattresses, 60
posture, 60
reading in bed, 61
seats, 61
sitting on floors, 60
sleeping position, 60
sport and, 60
weight and, 60
weight training and, 60, 66
Baths, after exercising, 9
Beans, recommended
servings, 75
Beds:
mattresses, 55, 60
reading in, 61
sleeping position, 60
Blood circulation:
aerobics and, 70
pregnancy and, 55
Bowel habits, 55
Breads, recommended
servins, 74
Breasts: *see* bust
Breathing:

exercises, *84, 85*
exercising and, 9
fitness and, 84-5
Bust:
exercises, 26-30
size increase, 86-7
Butter, 88
Buttock exercises, 36-9

C

Caffeine, pregnant
women, 55
Calorific values, 75
Cancer, fat and, 78
Cardiorespiratory
system:
aerobics and, 70
monitoring, 71
Carrying heavy objects, 60
lifting the object, 61, *61*
Cellulite, 87
Cereals, recommended
servings, 74
Chairs, backaches and, 61
Cheese, recommended
servings, 74
Chest exercises, 26-30
Cholesterol, 78
Cigarettes, 55
Circulation:
aerobics and, 70
pregnant women, 55
Classes, aerobic dance, 73
Clothes:
for exercising in, 9
running shoes, 72
socks, 72
walking shoes, 73
Cool-down exercises, 8, 50-4
Cramp, 55
Cream, non-dairy, 88
Cycling, *70*

D

Dancing, aerobic, *72,* 73
Diet:
dangers of, 77
dining with friends, 81

fiber, 76
healthy habits, 76, 77
restaurant dining, 80
see also food
Dining:
with friends, 81, *81*
restaurants, 80-1
see also food
Doctors, consulting, 9, 55, 86
Drinks, 9
sugary, 79

E

Eating:
dining out, 80-1
speed of, 76
see also food
Exercises:
aerobic, 70-3
back exercises, 62-4
benefits of, 6
breathing and, 9
bust exercises, 26-30
buttock exercises, 36-40
clothes for, 9
cool-downs, 8, 50-4
heartbeat and, 71
hip exercises, 16-20
main, 8
monitoring progress, 71
music for, 9
prenatal, 56-9
showers after, 9
slimming, 64-5
soreness and, 9
stomach exercises, 45-9
thigh exercises, 21-5
thirst and, 9
tips, 9
upper arm exercises, 31-5
ventilation and, 9
waist exercises, 41-4
warm-ups, 8, 10-15
weight training, 66-9
when to, 9
where to, 9